Craniofacial Disorders – Orofacial Features and Peculiarities in Dental Treatment

Edited by:

Gisele da Silva Dalben
&
Marcia Ribeiro Gomide

Pediatric Dentist, Hospital for Rehabilitation of Craniofacial Anomalies, University of São Paulo, Bauru, Brazil

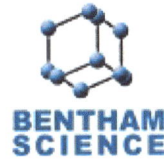

CONTENTS

FOREWORD 1

During my life I was assigned several missions: dentist, professor, researcher, manager; all of them were pleasant and full of challenges, with the bonus of knowing and living together with special people. I am proud to be invited to present this book to the world of Dentistry. The experience at the Hospital for Rehabilitation of Craniofacial Anomalies (HRAC-USP) gave me the opportunity to follow the career of several professionals, from undergraduate training up to the highest levels of research and university life. Few feelings are more thorough than following the personal and professional growth of people we respect; and the better reward for a professor is to see the shine of enthusiasm and curiosity in the eyes of young professionals, thirsty for knowledge; for a manager, to follow the vibration with which the team conducts its work. I have learned more than I have taught. At HRAC-USP, the daily routine was always filled with technical and human challenges. The daily care for individuals with different disabilities provides professionals with a rich source of research inspiration, besides demands yet to be explored. It is enough to be willing. The editors Gisele da Silva Dalben, Marcia Ribeiro Gomide and the contributor Beatriz Costa are examples of this thirst for knowledge and clinical sensitivity. They are three great researchers who were shaped at the Pediatric Dentistry clinic of HRAC/USP, where they sharpened and deepened their skills on the needs of patients requiring differentiated attention and treatment, respecting their exceptional birth conditions. Part of the long years of study, investigation and practice of these three brilliant researchers is present in this book, which surely enriches the dental management of patients with craniofacial anomalies. The book gathers experiences, knowledge and tips that the contributors kindly offer to anyone interested in this field. A part of their lives, all of them built inside Pediatric Dentistry. The years have been generous for me, giving me the opportunity to publicly celebrate the scientific maturity of three great pediatric dentists – and friends: Gisele, Marcia and Beatriz. And I say with certainty that another important chapter of Dentistry was written.

Dr. José Alberto de Souza Freitas ("Tio Gastão")
Founder and former superintendent of HRAC/USP,
Full Professor of University of São Paulo,
Brazil

FOREWORD 2

Writing the foreword to this book "Craniofacial disorders – orofacial features and peculiarities in dental treatment" has been a reason of great joy and pride, since this is one more contribution of the Hospital for Rehabilitation of Craniofacial Anomalies of University of São Paulo, gently known as "Centrinho", to the specialized literature.

Both editors are dental professionals graduated by FOB-USP with Master and PhD degrees and are extremely dedicated professionals who, together, add up more than 50 years of contribution to clinical activities, rehabilitating and providing smiles to individuals with craniofacial anomalies, besides actively working in the Teaching and Research scopes of the institution, valuing the scientific production.

The book is composed of nine chapters that bring valuable information for dentists and health professionals caring for individuals with syndromes associated with craniofacial anomalies. The book presents an update approach about Craniofacial Embryology, Concepts of Genetics, Teratogenesis, Dental Management in Rare Facial Clefts, as well as the alterations accompanying the diverse Syndromes with Orofacial Clefts, Craniosynostosis Syndromes, First Pharyngeal Arch Disorders, Syndromes with Characteristic Facies, and an approach about the Surgical Treatment in Craniofacial Malformations: Distraction Osteogenesis.

Further, the HRAC-USP has a strong team working on Genetics associated with craniofacial anomalies, coordinated by the medical geneticist Dr Antonio Richieri Costa, and during 50 years of work the institution concentrates a databank that is a scientific treasure. During her PhD, Dr Gisele da Silva Dalben worked with Dr Richieri Costa, analyzing individuals with Opitz G/BBB syndrome, and has several publications in the subject of craniofacial syndromes.

Since HRAC/USP is a reference center in craniofacial anomalies with participation of an interdisciplinary team, it was possible to prepare this book especially focusing the interest of dental professionals.

I consider this book a precious masterpiece, which shall fill the gap currently existing in the literature, concentrating in a single work the information on dental, skeletal and craniofacial alterations in individuals with different craniofacial disorders.

Dr. Terumi Okada Ozawa
Orthodontist and former Director of Dental Division of HRAC/USP,
Brazil

PREFACE

In 2003, the editors of this book noticed a lack of organized information about dental care for individuals with craniofacial disorders. Then, the editors performed a literature review about different craniofacial disorders and wrote an informal handout, which the editors made available in the local library. As years went by, that handout turned out to be widely borrowed and used as reference in their institution, which encouraged the editors to expand the information and transform that handout in the present ebook.

The editors work as pediatric dentists in a tertiary hospital and are often challenged with a wide array of disorders, frequently facing situations in which individuals and their families must travel even days to attend the institution for accomplishment of dental procedures that could be performed by professionals at their cities of origin, if only they had a little more information about craniofacial disorders. In some international experiences, the editors observed that, worldwide, there is still a lot of misconception and disinformation about when and how to treat the different disorders present in individuals with craniofacial disorders.

The organization of this book into chapters was largely based on the classic book "Syndromes of the head and neck" (Gorlin, 1990), which the editors consider fundamental for professionals who want to dive deeper into the world of craniofacial disorders.

To enhance the understanding on "hows and whys", Chapter 1 presents rich information about craniofacial embryology. This chapter was written by the eminent embryologist Kathleen K. Sulik, who describes craniofacial development in detail with the aid of amazing scanning electron micrographs of embryos, allowing the reader to travel through the stages of normal and abnormal embryonic development.

Chapters 2 and 3 present basic concepts of genetics and teratology, enhancing the knowledge of readers so that they can better understand the information presented in following chapters.

Chapters 4 to 8 describe the different craniofacial disorders in a similar sequence as in "Syndromes of the head and neck", presenting the disorders with their respective etiology, systemic involvement, and peculiarities in dental treatment. All contributors in these chapters have current and/or previous clinical experience in providing dental care to individuals with craniofacial malformations, and much of the information presented in these chapters were observed in investigations conducted at the editors' institution.

Finally, in Chapter 9, the authors describe the surgical steps required for complex dentomaxillofacial reconstruction in different disorders. These surgical procedures aim at both esthetic and functional improvement, and are paramount for the thorough rehabilitation of individuals.

The aim of this ebook is to be a chairside resource for clinical dentists who wish to offer dental care for individuals with craniofacial disorders. The editors' goal, when organizing this ebook, was to enhance the knowledge of dental professionals across the world about craniofacial disorders, their orodental features and peculiarities in dental treatment, so that individuals affected by such syndromes may have increasingly better and easier access to dental care.

We wish the readers all the best when assisting individuals with craniofacial malformations. We hope you will find the present information useful, and we wish you a rewarding experience in treating these individuals and watching them grow stronger and more self-reassured with your collaboration.

We also wish all the best to individuals with craniofacial malformations and their families, with special consideration to those attending the editors' institution – the Hospital for Rehabilitation of Craniofacial Anomalies, University of São Paulo at Bauru, Brazil, who were the main driving force behind this ebook, and special thanks to individuals and their families who kindly granted permission to publish their images in this ebook. This book was inspired by you, and is dedicated to you.

ACKNOWLEDGEMENT

Chapters 2 to 9 were originally written in Portuguese and translated into English by the author Gisele da Silva Dalben. Signed informed consent was obtained from all individuals whose facial photographs that allow their identification are presented in this ebook.

All photographs presented in Chapter 1 belong to the files of the chapter author. Photographs presented in Chapters 2 through 9 belong to the files from respective chapter authors, from the Hospital for Rehabilitation of Craniofacial Anomalies of University of São Paulo, and from Adriano Porto Peixoto, who kindly granted access to his files.

Gisele da Silva Dalben
Pediatric and Community Dentistry Sector,
Hospital for Rehabilitation of Craniofacial Anomalies,
University of São Paulo,
Bauru,
Brazil

&

Marcia Ribeiro Gomide
Pediatric and Community Dentistry Sector,
Hospital for Rehabilitation of Craniofacial Anomalies,
University of São Paulo,
Bauru,
Brazil

DEDICATION

To my dearest parents, Oswaldo and Madalena, who taught me everything that is important for a worthy life;
To my husband Maurício and my precious kids Lucas and Vitor, who make my life even worthier;
To the authors of chapters in this book, all of whom I consider outstanding professionals in their respective fields of work and lifelong companions in this amazing journey of caring for individuals with craniofacial malformations;
Above all, to the individuals with craniofacial malformations, especially those who kindly granted permission to publish their images herein, who teach us so much about the meaning of life and who are the main reason for writing this book.

Gisele da Silva Dalben

To my family, the place chosen by God for me in the world, where I learned, besides unconditional love, honesty with my father Nilton, faith with my mother Linda, fraternity with my brothers Mariângela, Mariza and Nilton, and endless happiness with my husband Wagner and my children Camila, Fernando, Rafael and Andressa.

Marcia Ribeiro Gomide

List of Contributors

Adriano Porto Peixoto Orthodontics and Dentofacial Orthopedics Sector and Craniofacial Surgery Sector Hospital for Rehabilitation of Craniofacial Anomalies, University of São Paulo, Bauru, Brazil

Ana Lúcia Pompéia Fraga de Almeida Department of Prosthodontics, Bauru School of Dentistry, University of São Paulo, Bauru, Brazil
Hospital for Rehabilitation of Craniofacial Anomalies, University of São Paulo, Bauru, Brazil

Beatriz Costa Pediatric and Community Dentistry Sector Hospital for Rehabilitation of Craniofacial Anomalies, University of São Paulo, Bauru, Brazil

Cleide Felício de Carvalho Carrara Pediatric and Community Dentistry Sector Hospital for Rehabilitation of Craniofacial Anomalies, University of São Paulo, Bauru, Brazil

Cristiano Tonello Craniofacial Surgery Sector Hospital for Rehabilitation of Craniofacial Anomalies, University of São Paulo, Bauru, Brazil

Gisele da Silva Dalben Pediatric and Community Dentistry Sector Hospital for Rehabilitation of Craniofacial Anomalies, University of São Paulo, Bauru, Brazil

Kathleen K. Sulik Bowles Center for Alcohol Studies School of Medicine, University of North Carolina, Chapel Hill, USA

Lucimara Teixeira das Neves Discipline of Genetics, Bauru School of Dentistry, University of São Paulo, Bauru, Brazil
Hospital for Rehabilitation of Craniofacial Anomalies, University of São Paulo, Bauru, Brazil

Marcia Ribeiro Gomide Pediatric and Community Dentistry Sector Hospital for Rehabilitation of Craniofacial Anomalies, University of São Paulo, Bauru, Brazil

Maurício Mitsuru Yoshida Craniofacial Surgery Sector (Former member) Hospital for Rehabilitation of Craniofacial Anomalies, University of São Paulo, Bauru, Brazil
Santa Marcelina Hospital, São Paulo, Brazil
Medical School of ABC, Santo André, Brazil

Melissa Zattoni Antonelli Speech-Language Pathology Sector Hospital for Rehabilitation of Craniofacial Anomalies, University of São Paulo, Bauru, Brazil

Michele Madeira Brandão Craniofacial Surgery Sector Hospital for Rehabilitation of Craniofacial AnomaliesUniversity of São Paulo, Bauru, Brazil

Nivaldo Alonso Medical School, University of São Paulo, São Paulo, Brazil
Craniofacial Surgery Sector Hospital for Rehabilitation of Craniofacial Anomalies, University of São Paulo, Bauru, Brazil

Vivian de Agostino Biella Passos School of Dentistry, University of Sagrado Coração, Bauru, Brazil

Glossary

- Anophthalmia – absence of eye formation

- Anotia – absence of ear formation

- Arachnodactyly – condition in which the fingers are long, thin and curved, resembling the legs of a spider

- Blepharophimosis – combination of small eyelids, reduced palpebral opening, telecanthus, ptosis, arched eyebrows and epicanthal folds

- Brachydactyly – shortening of digits

- Camptodactyly – deformity caused by flexure of the proximal interphalangeal joint, usually of the fifth finger

- Clinodactyly – arched digits

- Coloboma – congenital fissure of any structure of the eye

- Craniosynostosis – premature closure of cranial sutures

- Cryptorchidism – absence of the testicles in the scrotum due to persistence inside the abdomen or inguinal canal

- Dysostosis – defect in ossification

- Dysplasia – abnormal development of organs and tissues causing deformities

- Ectrodactyly – congenital absence of one or more fingers or toes

- Ectropium – eversion of an edge or margin, usually of the eyelid

- Encephalocele – hernia of the brain or cerebellum through a congenital or traumatic opening in the skull

- Etiology – investigation of the causes of a disease

- Exotropia – strabismus in which the eye is directed outwards

- Extrophy – congenital eversion of an organ or part of it

- Glossoptosis – tongue retraction

- Hyperteleorbitism – increased distance between the orbits

- Hypertelorism – increased distance between any two symmetric structures in the body

- Hypoteleorbitism – reduced distance between the orbits

- Hypoacusia – reduced hearing ability

- Hypogonadism – inadequate gonadal function, manifested by deficiency in gametogenesis and/or secretion of gonadal hormones

- Hypohidrosis – reduction of sweat

- Hypospadia – congenital and abnormal opening of the urethra on the inferior part of the penis. It may also affect females, leading the urine to flow through the vagina

- Lagophthalmos – paralysis of an eyelid precluding complete closure of the eye globe when closed

- Meningomyelocele – hernia of part of the spinal cord and its meninges

- Microbrachycephaly – reduction and shortening of head size
- Microcephaly – reduction of head size
- Microphthalmia – reduction of eye size
- Microtia – reduction of ear size
- Nystagmus – fast and involuntary oscillation of the eye globe around its horizontal or vertical axis
- Oligodactyly – reduction in the number of fingers or toes
- Oligohydramnios – significant reduction in amniotic fluid volume
- Pectus excavatum – depression or groove caused by more interior positioning of the sternum
- Polydactyly – increase in the number of fingers or toes
- Polyhydramnios – significant increase in amniotic fluid volume
- Epicanthal fold – skin fold in the internal eye canthus, displacing the upper eyelid toward the internal canthus
- Proptosis – anterior displacement, usually of the eye
- Syndactyly – congenital union between one or more fingers or toes
- Synophrys – conjunction of the eyebrows
- Telecanthus – increased distance between the internal eye canthi, caused by lateral displacement of the medial canthus

CHAPTER 1

Normal and Abnormal Oro-Facial Embryogenesis

Kathleen K. Sulik[1,*]

[1] *Bowles Center for Alcohol Studies, School of Medicine, University of North Carolina, Chapel Hill, USA*

Abstract: The focus of this chapter is on normal oro-facial embryogenesis; on the developmental basis for facial defects that fall within the holoprosencephaly spectrum; and on the genesis of common and unusual oro-facial clefts. A thorough understanding of normal morphogenesis coupled with appreciation of the dysmorphogenic events underlying the defects considered in this chapter should aid the reader in also better appreciating the developmental basis for many of the other abnormalities addressed in this text. The prenatal stages considered in detail are present from the 3rd through the 8th weeks of human gestation, with emphasis being placed on description of the development of the growth centers (prominences/processes) that comprise the human oro-facies. The presence and significance of some of these oro-facial growth centers for both normal and abnormal embryogenesis have been largely overlooked in the past, due in part to the paucity of early human embryos available for careful analyses with modern techniques. To aid in resolving this problem, descriptions provided herein are largely founded on a relatively recent series of scanning electron micrographs of human embryos. Regarding clefting, knowledge of normal oro-facial morphogenesis, coupled with basic research findings, support the premise that the junctions of the various growth centers correspond to the sites of common and unusual oro-facial clefts as described by Tessier in 1976 [45]; that the embryonic period is when the vast majority of oro-facial clefts are induced; and that, in most cases, the proximate cause of clefting is failure of the normal growth and development of single or adjacent oro-facial growth centers. As for holoprosencephaly, both genetic abnormalities and environmental insults can underlie the dysmorphology.

Keywords: Cleft lip, Cleft palate, Embryology, Holoprosencephaly, Malformation, Oro-facial, Unusual facial cleft.

INTRODUCTION

An understanding of normal oro-facial embryogenesis is key to appreciation of the genesis of malformations involving this region. To facilitate learning, in this chapter scanning electron microscopic images of normal early human embryos are utilized as the primary tool to illustrate the complex changes in form that occur

---

* Corresponding author Kathleen K. Sulik: Bowles Center for Alcohol Studies, School of Medicine, University of North Carolina, Chapel Hill, United States of America; Tel/Fax: +1 (919) 966-5678; E-mail: mouse@med.unc.edu

Gisele da Silva Dalben & Marcia Ribeiro Gomide (Eds.)

during the 1st trimester of gestation. With much of our knowledge regarding embryonic development having been acquired from the study of normal, mutant, and teratogen-treated non-human animals, pertinent animal images and research findings are also included. With a few exceptions as noted herein, the images are from the author's collection; human embryos having been collected by Dr. Michel Vekemans and Tania Attie-Bitacha, Necker Hospital, Paris, France. Cellular events underlying normal oro-facial embryogenesis will be addressed briefly as will developmental events that are pertinent to the generation of facial defects present in the holoprosencephaly (HPE) spectrum and that result in oro-facial clefts. Emphasis is placed on description of the morphogenesis of distinct growth centers of the developing face, on their apparent segmental nature, and on the correspondence of these growth centers and failures of their development, fusion or merging to the majority of the recognized oro-facial clefting sites as defined by Tessier [1]. A thorough understanding of normal morphogenesis coupled with appreciation of the dysmorphogenic events underlying the defects considered in this chapter should aid the reader in also better appreciating the developmental basis for many of the other abnormalities addressed in this text. For more comprehensive instruction, readers are referred to current embryology textbooks and web sites and also to recent review articles [2 - 12].

With the objective of providing the reader a broad perspective on the remarkable developmental changes involved in oro-facial embryogenesis, Fig. (**1.1**) illustrates the developmental progression that occurs from the human 3rd through 8th week post-fertilization [Please note that all age references are to days post-fertilization as opposed to post-last normal menstrual period]. During this 6-week span of time the embryo transitions from having a disk-like shape of only 0.5 mm in diameter to having a fetal form with a crown-rump length of approximately 3 cm. The end of the 8th week after fertilization is considered the end of the embryonic period and the beginning of the fetal period of prenatal life. While the secondary palate closes early in the 9th week and, therefore remains vulnerable to cleft-inducing insult during the early fetal stages, the vast majority of oro-facial clefts, as well as the HPE spectrum and defects including some forms of micrognathia and many ocular and auricular malformations are induced during the embryonic period.

Because the earliest of the developmental stages considered are likely the most unfamiliar/least intuitive to most readers, the majority of the images in Fig. (**1.1**) are of 3 and 4-week-old embryos. For the 3-week-old embryos, both light and scanning electron microscopic images are shown, illustrating the greater surface detail evident in the latter. The 3rd week is marked by neural plate formation and the ventral growth/folding of the embryo that creates a foregut pocket dorsal to the developing heart. In the 4th week, the neural tube closes and the pharyngeal (branchial; visceral) arches become evident. The olfactory placodes, around which the nose will form, become apparent in the 5th week. And, from the 6th through the 8th weeks the various growth centers/facial prominences surrounding the nose, mouth, and eyes remodel as the face acquires a recognizably human appearance.

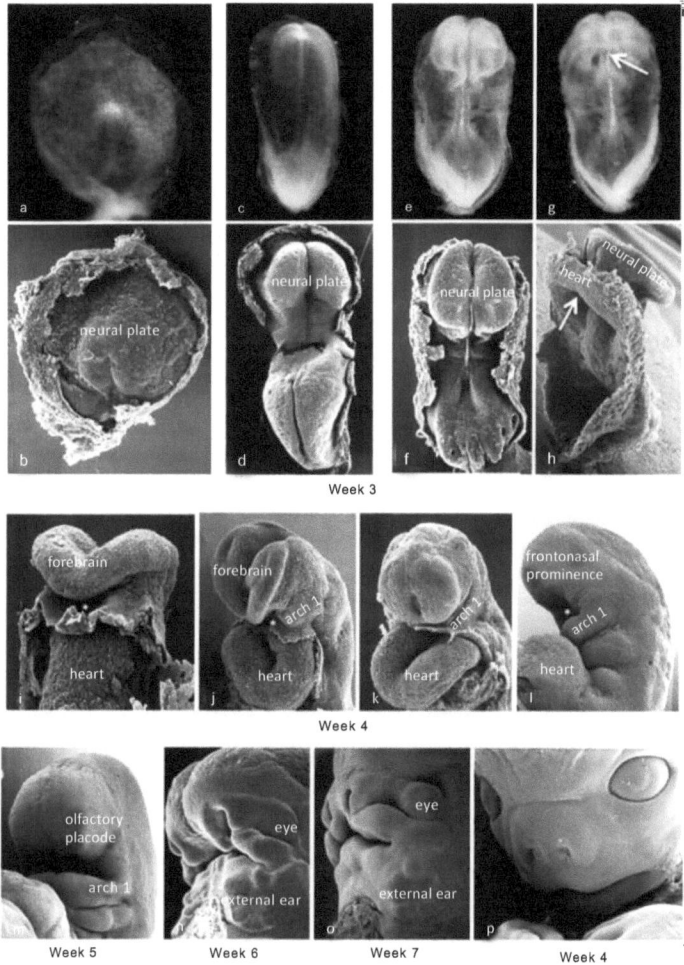

Fig. (1.1). A succession of stages of human embryonic development is shown in light micrographs (a, c, e, g) and scanning electron micrographs (b, d, f, h-p). Approximate ages for each of the embryos shown are as follows: 17 days (a, b), 19 days (c, d), 21 days (e-h), 23 days (i), 24 days (j), 25 days (k), 26 days (l), 32 days (m); 41 days (n); 43 days (o), 52 days (p). Views shown in (a-f) are dorsal; (g) is a ventral view; and (h-p) are ventrolateral views. Arrow in (g, h) = foregut; * = stomodeum (primitive oral cavity). (n) is reprinted from Hinrichsen [13].

NORMAL ORO-FACIAL EMBRYOGENESIS

While the first 2 weeks after fertilization are marked by the initial cell divisions and interactions from which the embryo and its supporting tissues are generated, it is in the 3rd week that all 3 of the embryos' definitive germ layers (the ectoderm, mesoderm, and endoderm) are established. The ectoderm covers the dorsal surface of the embryo; the endoderm the ventral surface; and the mesoderm fills the majority of the space in between the other 2 cell layers. This is illustrated in Fig. (**1.2**) which is comprised of dorsal (Fig. **1.2a, b**) and ventral (Fig. **1.2d-f**) views of the 19 day old, approximately 2 mm long embryo previously shown in Fig. (**1.1c, d**), along with a cross-sectional view of a comparably-staged mouse embryo (Fig. **1.2c**). As readily seen in the latter, at this stage of development, the ectodermal cells have a columnar shape, the endodermal cells are more flattened (squamous), and the mesodermal cells have a fibroblastic morphology. In the rostral midline, there are only 2 layers of cells, with the ventral cells of this bilayer making up the prechordal and notochordal plates. Cells comprising the prechordal plate underlie the developing forebrain and produce molecular signals that are critical to normal forebrain development. Further caudally, on the ventral aspect of the embryo is a specialized population of cells that have long (approximately 2 microns), motile monocilia (Fig. **1.2e, f**). These (nodal) cilia were discovered in 1994 in a study of mouse embryos [14] and have subsequently been shown to generate a leftward flow of extracellular fluids; a phenomenon that is important in establishing the body's right-left asymmetry [15 - 17].

By the time the human embryo reaches the end of its 3rd week of development, 2 subpopulations of ectoderm can be readily distinguished: the surface and neural ectoderm. As shown in Fig. (**1.3a**), the surface ectoderm covers the outer surface of the developing oro-facies, including the stomodeum (primitive oral cavity). Prior to neural tube closure, the surface and neural ectoderm are continuous, the latter being the source of the central nervous system. The dashed line in Fig. (**1.3a**) is at the surface/neural ectodermal junction. For the oro-facies, a population of neural ectoderm-derived cells termed neural crest gives rise to the skeletal and other connective tissues (except tooth enamel), as well as to cranial ganglia neurons, smooth muscle of the skin, ciliary muscles, meninges, Schwann cells and melanocytes. In Fig. (**1.3b**), an image made following a cut through the rostral-most aspect of a mouse embryo of the same developmental stage as the human in Fig. (**1.3a**) shows emigrating neural crest cells at the margin of the neural plate. In addition to neural crest cells, mesodermal cells populate the developing oro-facies, the latter serving as the source of striated muscle. While not readily seen nor shown herein, the mesodermal cells that are adjacent to the neural plate are segmented into aggregates of cells termed somitomeres that are in consistent relationship with the segments of the developing brain and face and that contribute the myoblasts for specific facial muscles [18 - 20]. The endoderm which lines the developing gut (the most rostral component of which is the oropharyngeal portion of the foregut) gives rise to the parenchyma of glandular structures including the tonsils and thymus. The relationship between the ectoderm, mesoderm and endoderm is also illustrated in Fig. (**1.3c**), which shows a mouse embryo cut in a parasagittal plane. Notable is that, with the cut through this embryo not being midsagittal, the buccopharyngeal membrane, which is a midline structure formed by apposition of the stomodeal (primitive oral cavity) surface ectoderm and the pharyngeal endoderm, is not evident (see Fig. (**1.7**) for an image of the buccopharyngeal membrane). Instead, at the level of this cut, mesoderm separates these cell layers (see boxed area in Fig. (**1.3c**)).

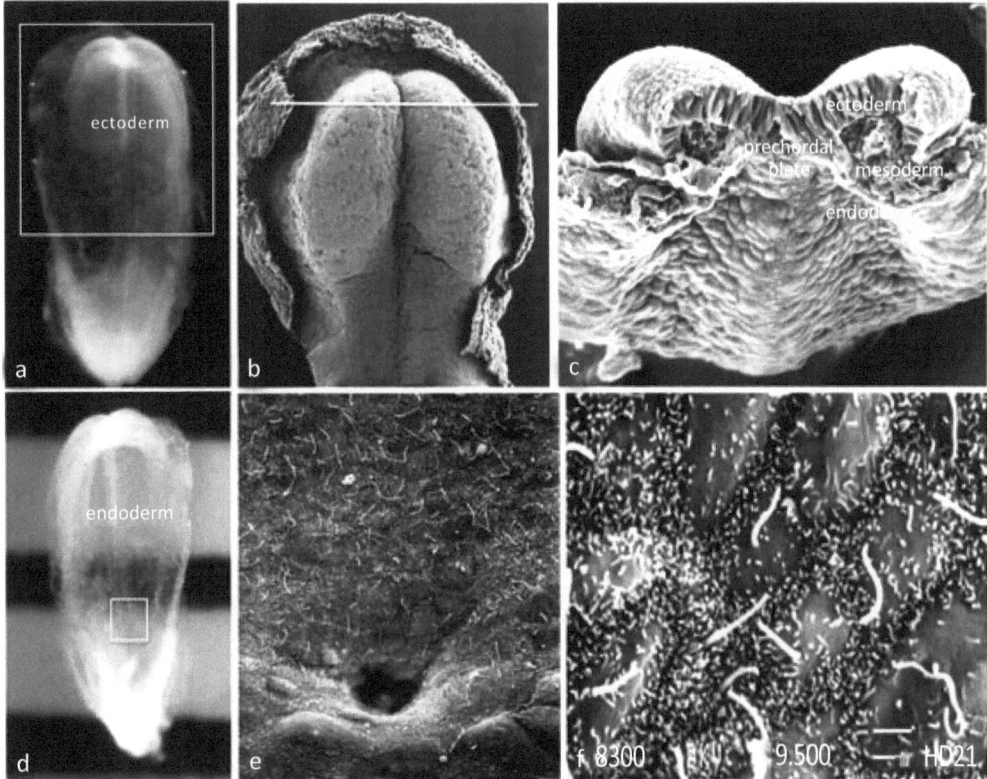

Fig. (1.2). Dorsal (a, b) and ventral (d-f) views of a 19 day old human embryo and a cross-sectional view of a comparably staged mouse embryo (c) illustrate the germ layers; ectoderm, mesoderm, and endoderm. Shown in (c) is the mesoderm and the prechordal plate which underlies the developing forebrain. The line in (b) = level of section for (c). A specialized population of cells having motile monocilia is located at the level of the boxed area in (d) and is shown at increasingly higher magnification in (e) and (f), respectively.

By the time the human embryo enters its 4th week of development, it is approximately 3 mm long, with the developing head and neck making up half of the length (Fig. **1.4**). A dorsal view shows that, while the dorsal aspect of the neural folds are closely opposed at the level of the junction between the developing brain and spinal cord [arrow in (a)], fusion to form the neural tube has not yet begun. Sub-segments of the developing brain are evident at this developmental stage; the segments from rostral to caudal being termed the forebrain (prosencephalon) midbrain (mesencephalon) and hindbrain (rhombencephalon). These 3 major brain segments are further subdivided into neuromeres, with the hindbrain having 8 that are termed rhombomeres, the midbrain having 2 mesomeres, and the prosencephalon being subdivided into a diencephalic portion that is comprised of 3 prosomeres and into a telencephalic portion (also referred to as the secondary prosencephalon; and that appears to also have 3 prosomeric subdivisions). The telencephalon has a dorsal component from which the cerebral hemispheres arise and a ventral, hypothalamic, component [21, 22] (also see Fig. (**1.9**)). With the segments of the developing brain being in register with those of the face and neck, appreciating their presence and position is particularly important. An example of this brain/face relationship that can be seen in Fig. (**1.4**) is that the developing 1ˢᵗ pharyngeal arch is aligned with the neuromeres of the lower midbrain (mesomere 2) and upper hindbrain (rhombomeres 1 and 2). The lateral margins of these neuromeres are the source of the neural crest cells that populate the 1ˢᵗ arch-derived regions. Notably, the margin of the diencephalon is generally considered to be the rostral-most source of neural crest cells; most experimental studies indicating that none come from the margin of the telencephalon.

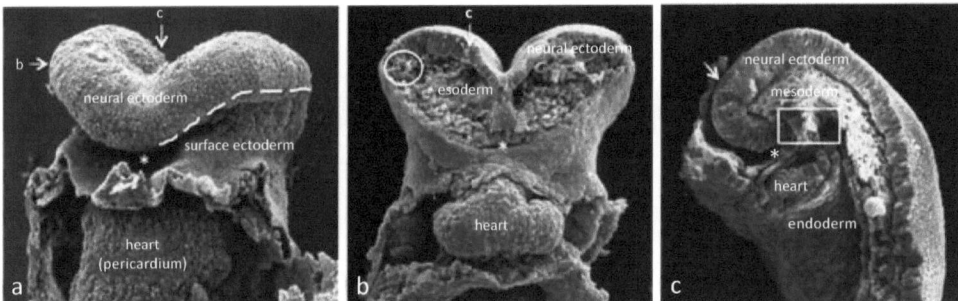

Fig. (1.3). Images of the oro-facial region of a human embryo at the end of the 3ʳᵈ week (a) and of 2 comparably staged mouse embryos (b, c) illustrate the relationship between the ectoderm, mesoderm, and endoderm and the formation of the stomodeum (primitive oral cavity). Arrows = the plane of section for images shown in (b, c); dashed line = junction between neural and surface ectoderm; circle = neural crest cells; box indicates 3 germ layers located just lateral to the buccopharyngeal membrane; * = stomodeum.

Neural fold fusion/neural tube closure occurs during the 4ᵗʰ week after fertilization, being initiated at cervical levels and progressing in both cranial (rostral) and caudal directions. It is notable that as cranial neural tube closure reaches midbrain levels, the lateral margins of the developing forebrain fold medially, allowing their union in the midline (Fig. **1.5**). The rostral progression of closure is accompanied by a relatively short span of union that extends dorsally from the ventral-most aspect of the forebrain. The final site of cranial (anterior neuropore) closure is near the junction of the telencephalic and diencephalic portions of the forebrain. Anterior neuropore closure is normally complete by 25 days after fertilization.

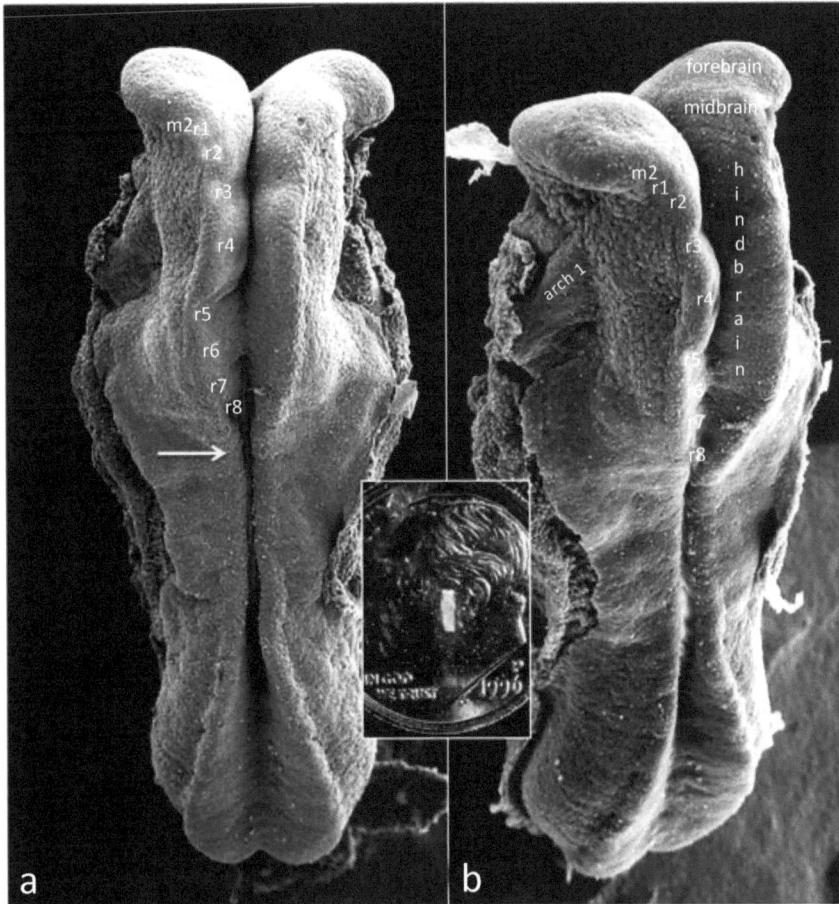

Fig. (1.4). Dorsal (a) and dorso-lateral (b) scanning electron microscopic views of a 22-day human embryo, along with placement on a US dime to illustrate relative size (approximately 3 mm). Arrow = junction between the developing brain and spinal cord and the approximate site of initial neural fold fusion. The position of the lower mesencephalic segment (mesomere 2; m2) and the rhombencephalic segments (r1-8) are shown. Note the spatial relationship between the 1st arch and the neural segments (m2, r1, r2) from which its neural crest cells originate.

At the developmental stages shown in Fig. (**1.5**) (and even earlier for rostral-most populations), neural crest cells emigrate from the margins of the neural folds to populate the developing face and neck. It appears that the cranial neural crest cells reach their destinations in part by being left behind as the neural folds elevate during closure, and in part through active migration [21, 23]. As previously noted, specific neural segments give rise to neural crest cells that populate defined regions. Fundamental to the segmental nature of craniofacial patterning is that there is very little intermixing between neural crest cell migratory streams [9]. As illustrated in Fig. (**1.6**), the neural crest cells that populate the frontonasal prominence (the tissue surrounding the forebrain) appear to arise from diencephalic and upper midbrain levels; those of the maxillary prominence arise from upper midbrain levels; those of the 1st pharyngeal arch arise from lower midbrain and upper hindbrain levels; and those of the more caudal arches come from correspondingly more caudal hindbrain regions [9, 12].

At the stage shown in Fig. (**1.6**), *i.e.* by the time of anterior neuropore closure, neural crest cells in the developing facial region are likely to have already reached their destinations. Also likely (though to the knowledge of the author, as yet unexplored experimentally) is that, as at more caudal levels, the neural crest cells emigrating from diencephalic levels do so in a segmental fashion consistent with the 3 diencephalic prosomeres; *i.e.* as segmental aggregates or streams. It is likely that interference with the normal genesis of specific rostral neural crest aggregates/streams is the basis for many of the recognized types of oro-facial clefts; a premise further discussed in the abnormal embryogenesis section below.

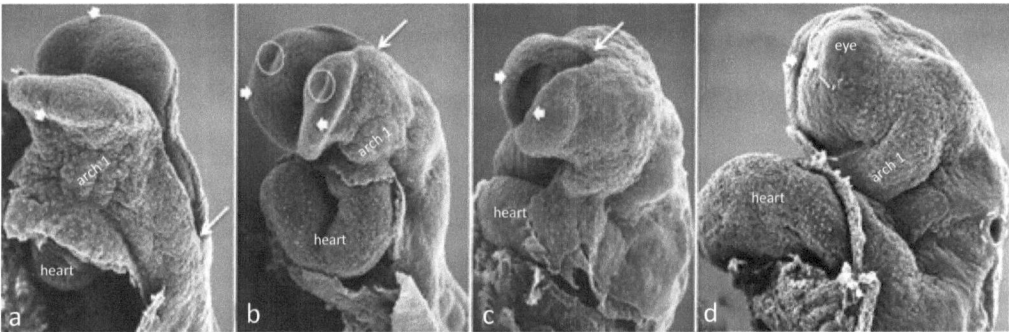

Fig. (1.5). Cranial neural tube closure occurs in the 4th week and should be complete by 25 days after fertilization. Approximate ages for each of the embryos shown are as follows: 23 days (a), 24 days (b), 24 days (c), 25 days (d). Arrow = cranial neural tube closure progression; block arrowhead = telencephalon/diencephalon junction; circles in (b) = optic pits/sulci (developing eyes); dashed circle in (d) = otic pit (developing inner ear).

The time of anterior neuropore closure is also when the buccopharyngeal membrane breaks down to allow continuity between the stomodeum (primitive oral cavity) and oropharynx (Fig. **1.7**). This membrane is comprised of surface ectoderm on the stomodeal side and endoderm on the pharyngeal side. Membranes consisting of surface ectoderm opposed to pharyngeal endoderm also are present between adjacent pharyngeal arches and are termed closing membranes. Closing membranes separate the pharyngeal clefts (external grooves between the arches) from the pharyngeal pouches (internal grooves between the arches). In some species the closing membranes normally break down, but this is not the case in humans.

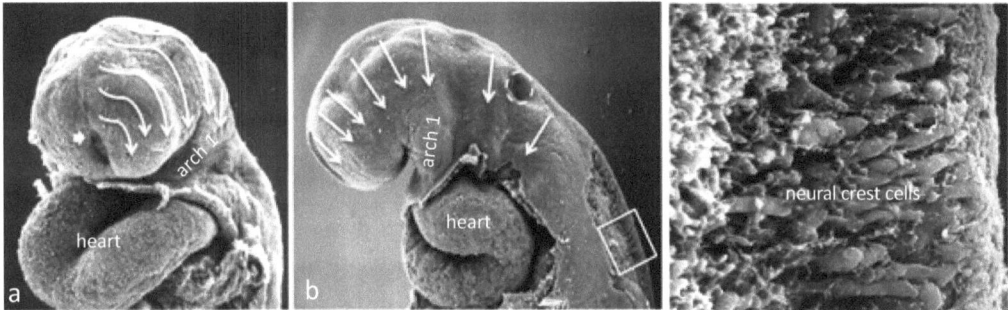

Fig. (1.6). Neural crest cells populate the developing face and neck, emigrating from the junction of neural and surface ectoderm at levels corresponding to specific segments of the developing brain (arrows). The embryo shown in both frontal (a) and lateral views (b, c; these images are flipped horizontally) is 25 days old. Notable is that at this stage, neural crest cells in the developing facial region are likely to have already reached their destinations and to have done so in a segmental fashion. The boxed area in (b) is shown at higher magnification in (c) and shows a region from which the surface ectoderm has been removed to reveal the subjacent neural crest cells that are leaving the dorsal aspect of the cervical neural tube. Block arrowhead in (a) = telencephalon/diencephalon junction; dashed circle in (b) = optic pit.

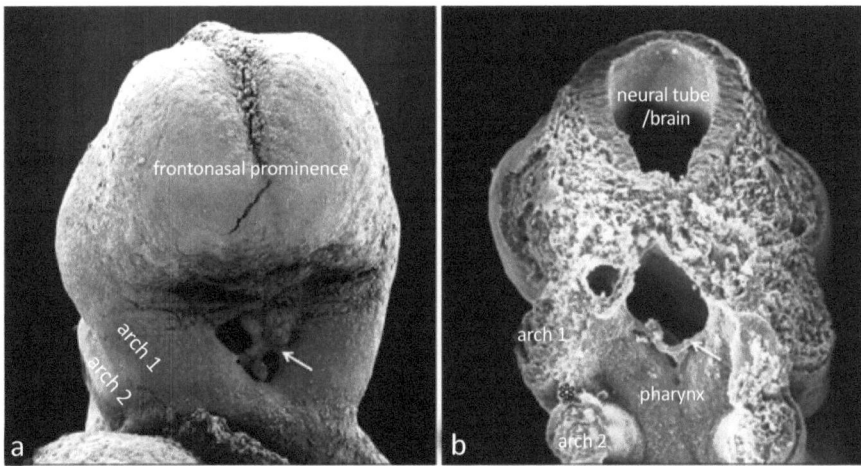

Fig. (1.7). Breakdown of the buccopharyngeal membrane allows continuity between the stomodeum and pharynx. The embryo in (a) is a 26-day human, while that in (b) is a mouse of a comparable developmental stage that has been cut and positioned to show the interior of the pharynx. Arrow = remnants of the buccopharyngeal membrane; * = the closing membrane between the 1st and 2nd pharyngeal arches; this membrane separates the 1st pharyngeal cleft (externally) and pouch (internally).

By the end of the 4th, to beginning of the 5th week, the developing oral cavity is bounded superiorly by the frontonasal prominence, superolaterally by distinct maxillary prominences/growth centers, and inferiorly by the 1st pharyngeal arches (Fig. **1.8**). The inferior boundary of the oral cavity has a prominent central notch between the bilateral 1st arch tissues. Additionally evident are the 2nd and 3rd pharyngeal arches with their corresponding clefts and pouches. The frontonasal prominence, which envelops the forebrain, has bilateral nasal placodes (thickened surface ectoderm) on its surface. As illustrated in Fig. (**1.8**), extending from the forebrain is the optic stalk and developing eye. Associated with the dorsal/proximal aspect of the maxillary prominence and 1st arch is the bulging trigeminal ganglion, which contains the sensory neurons for the face. These neurons have a dual origin; some of them being derived from neural crest cells while others originate from thickened surface ectoderm that forms a placode at the distal aspect of the developing ganglion. The position of this trigeminal placode as well as of other pharyngeal arch-related sensory (epibranchial) placodes is shown in Fig. (**1.9**).

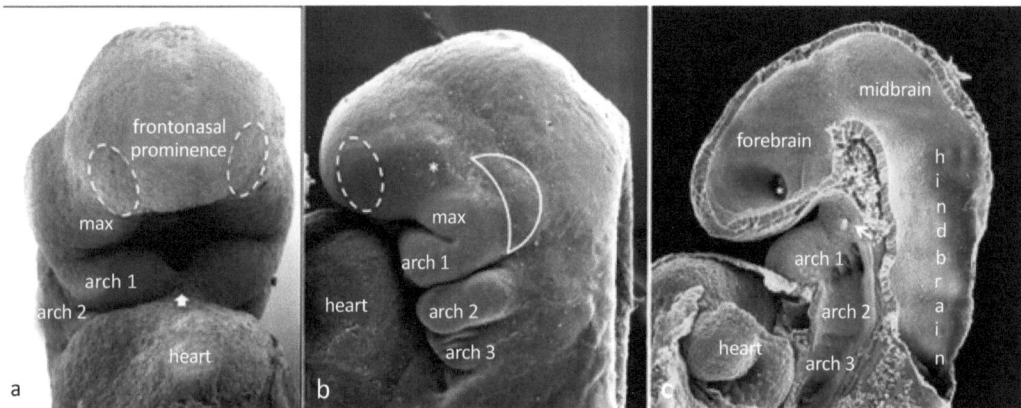

Fig. (1.8). Human embryos at 27 and 31 days post fertilization, respectively, are shown in (a) and (b). A correspondingly staged mouse embryo cut midsagittally is shown in (c). At this time, olfactory placodes (dashed circles) are visible on the surface of the frontonasal prominence, the latter of which envelops the forebrain. Notable are a deep central notch between the 1st arches (block arrowhead in a); a bulge created by the trigeminal ganglion (solid crescent in b) and by the developing eye (* in b); the optic stalk (* in c); and a remnant of the buccopharyngeal membrane (arrow in c). max = maxillary prominence/growth center.

Also shown in Fig. (**1.9**) are the contours of the developing brain, including the 3 prosomeres of the diencephalon which are evident even at the light microscopic level. The human embryo in this figure is in the middle of its 5th week of development; a time when the upper limb is paddle-shaped, having not yet developed digits, and when the dorsal aspect of the hindbrain region (*i.e.* the region of the 4th ventricle of the brain) is very thin-walled and appears relatively transparent.

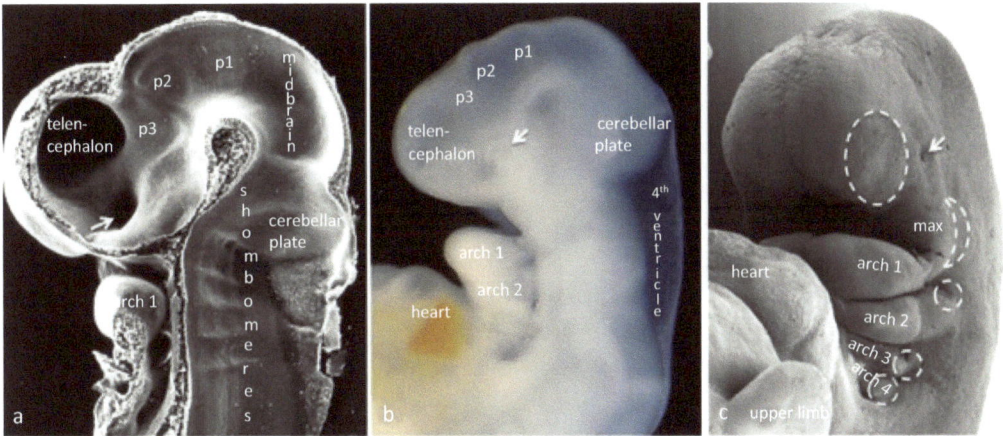

Fig. (1.9). A midsagittal cut through the head of a mouse embryo (a) along with a light micrograph (b) and scanning electron micrograph (c) of a 32-day human embryo illustrate the position of the optic stalk (arrow in a), eye (arrow in b) and lens pit (arrow in c), the sensory (olfactory, trigeminal, and epibranchial) placodes (dashed enclosures), and pharyngeal arches 1-4. Also, apparent at this developmental stage are the 3 segments of the diencephalon (prosomeres 1, 2, and 3; p1, p2, p3). max = maxillary prominence/growth center.

Progressing from the 5th to the 6th week of human development, the contours of the developing face become more complex as a number of growth centers become distinct. While described over 50 years ago [24], some of these growth centers (which appear as the surface bulges, processes, or prominences of the developing face) are not commonly noted in embryology texts. This failure has, undoubtedly, made the embryogenesis of unusual facial clefting sites difficult to understand. As shown in Figs. (**1.10 and 1.11**), the nasal pits become surrounded by tissue elevations termed the medial and lateral nasal prominences, both of which have 2 distinct growth centers; the dorsal (superior) portions are termed the *mnp* and *lnp*, respectively, while the respective ventral (inferior) portions are the premaxillary center (*premax*; also known as the Globular Process of His) and *lnp'*. Associated with the maxillary prominence (*max*) is a more rostrally located *max'*. Comprising the 1st arch are growth centers that contribute to the mentum (*man'*), to the remainder of the mandible (*man*), to the posterior-most aspect of the maxilla (*postmax*), and to the zygomaticotemporal region (*zt*). There are additional 1st arch growth centers that, along with growth centers in the 2nd arch (auricular hillocks), form the external ear.

While many sources continue to include the *max* growth center as part of the 1st arch, experimental analyses employing a chick model have shown it to be a separate entity [25]. As further discussed in the section on abnormal oro-facial embryogenesis, below, human embryo morphology and the position of typical clefting sites are consistent with the *max* growth center giving rise to the anterior portion of the maxilla, with the more posterior/caudal *postmax* tissues that are 1st

arch derivatives appearing to be the source of the posterior maxilla.

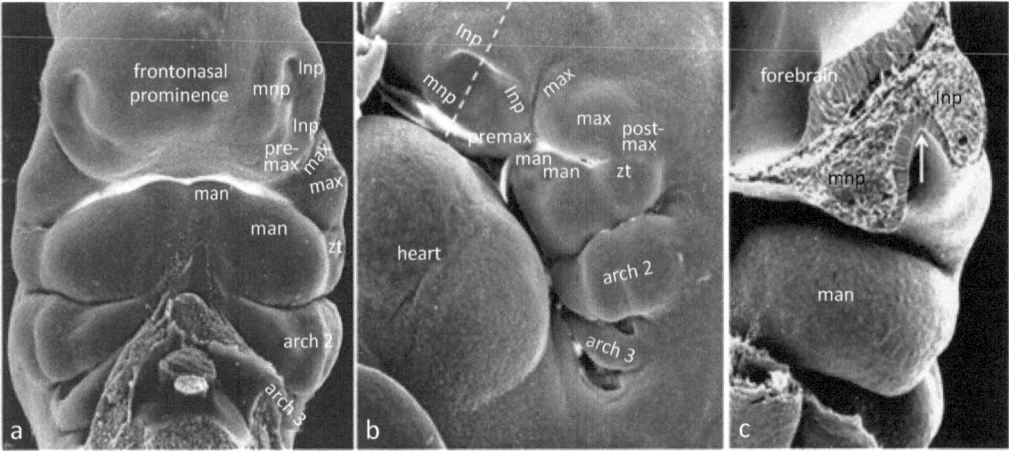

Fig. (1.10). By the middle of the 6th week, the human face develops a number of distinct growth centers/prominences as shown in frontal (a) and lateral (b) views. Included are those centers that surround the nasal pits and that are termed the medial and lateral nasal prominences, both of which have 2 components (mnp and premax; lnp and lnp'). There are two components of the maxillary region (max and max') and 4 facial components of the 1st arch (postmax, man', man, and zt). Shown in a cross section made at the level of the dashed line in (b) is a comparably staged mouse embryo (c). The olfactory placode (thickened surface ectoderm; arrow in c) lines the mnp and lnp-rimmed nasal pit.

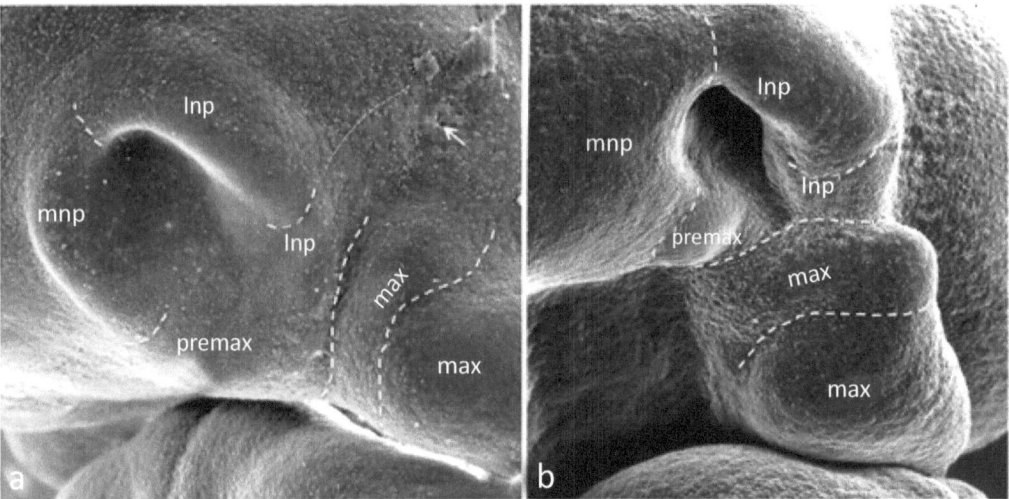

Fig. (1.11). The multiple growth centers of the developing face are illustrated in ventro-lateral views of a human (a) and a chick (b) embryo. Arrow = lens pit; premax = premaxillary prominence; mnp = medial nasal prominence; lnp = lateral nasal prominence; lnp' = lateral nasal prominence '; max' = maxillary prominence ' ; max = maxillary prominence.

As illustrated in Fig. (**1.11**), the facial growth centers/prominences in humans and non-human species are comparable. This is exemplified by the similar morphology of the nasal and maxillary region of a human embryo (the same embryo as in Fig. (**1.10**), but shown at higher magnification and at a ventro-lateral angle) and that of a comparably staged chick embryo. Distinction between each of the aforementioned growth centers is readily made. Additionally, notable is the relationship of *lnp'* and *max'* to the developing eye, the center of which is marked by the presence of the lens pit.

Closure of the upper lip occurs during the 6th week of human development. As shown in Fig. (**1.12**), which is comprised of a frontal view of a chick embryo along with a view of the roof of the oro-nasal cavity of a mouse embryo from which the lower jaw has been removed, lip closure is initiated with union of *lnp'* with the *premax* growth center bilaterally. Subsequently, *max'* also unites with the *premax*. Removal of the lower jaw reveals the medial extent of *max'* and *max*, both of which contribute to the upper alveolar ridge. Also notable is that at this developmental stage the space inside the nasal pit is not continuous with that of the inside of the mouth. The obstructing oro-nasal membrane later breaks down as shown in the Fig. (**1.12**) (b; inset), opening the primary choana. Just medial to the latter, and continuous anteriorly with the *premax*, is the tissue of the developing nasal septum.

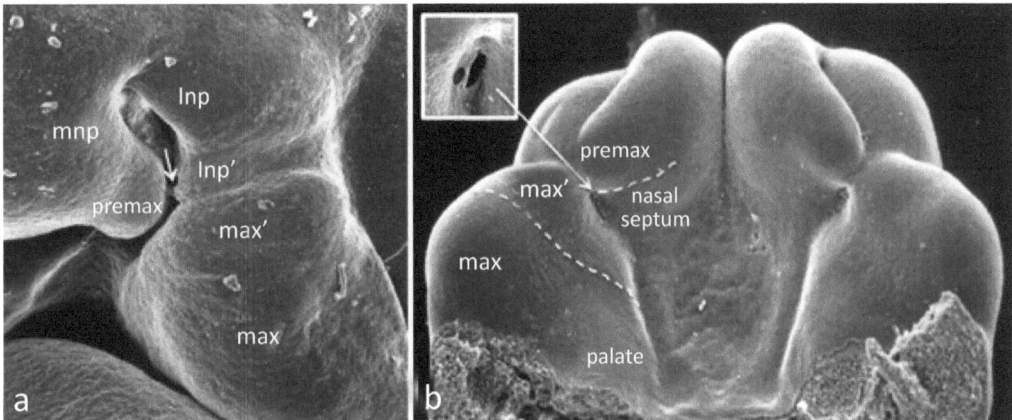

Fig. (1.12). As shown in chick (a) and mouse (b) embryos, bilateral union of lnp' with the premax (arrow in a), followed by union of max' with the premax (b) closes the upper lip. Extending medially to contribute to the alveolar ridges is tissue associated with both max' and max (b). These growth centers are shown separated by a dashed line in (b). The location of the oro-nasal membrane is indicated by the arrow in (b) and is shown in the inset at a later stage, when it is breaking down to create a patent primary choana.

Fig. (**1.13**) shows the face of a human embryo as it enters the 7th week post-fertilization, a time when the boundaries between the previously described facial growth centers remain relatively well delineated. While the upper lip is fused bilaterally, a prominent median groove remains between the *premax* centers. The 1st arch growth centers, including *man'* in the region of the mentum, *man*, and *zt*, remain evident and the auricular hillocks become more defined. Those that will form the tragus (1), crus (2), and anterior portion of the helix (3) of the external ear are part of the 1st arch tissue. The 2nd arch also contributes to the external ear as well as to the hyoid region of the neck. At this stage of development, eyelids have not yet formed and the eyes are laterally positioned relative to their definitive location.

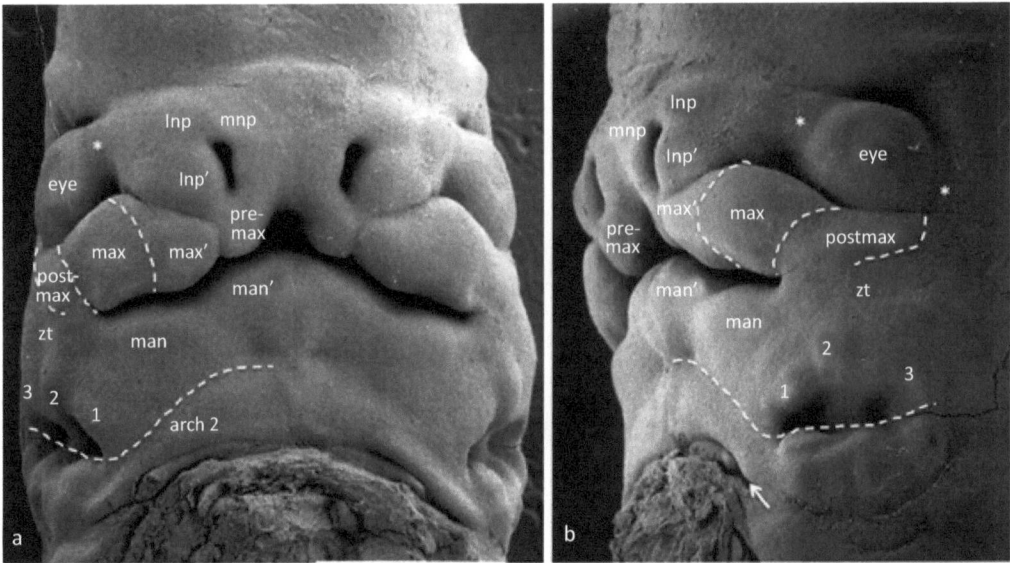

Fig. (1.13). Frontal (a) and front-lateral (b) views of an early 7th week (43 day) human embryo illustrate the facial growth centers. Dashed lines = the boundary of max and the boundary between 1st and 2nd arch tissues; the arrow in (b) points to the cervical sinus; * = medial and lateral canthal areas.

Continuing development in the 7th week, results in merging of the bilateral *premax* centers and smoothing of the contour of the upper lip margin. The *premax* contributes to the primary palate, the portion of the alveolar ridge containing the upper central incisors as well as the medial portion of the lateral incisors, and to the philtrum of the upper lip. While the boundaries between many of the facial growth centers are becoming indistinct at this time in development, those between the *premax*-derived philtrum and *max'*, and between *max'* and *max* remain apparent both on the facial and oral surfaces as shown in Fig. (**1.14**). Also evident in Fig. (**1.14**) is that the *max'* growth center contributes the facial/upper lip tissue that is located inferior to *lnp'*, the latter forming the inferior margin of the nostril. In addition to their contribution to the upper lip, the *max'* centers form the portion of the alveolar ridge that contains the primordia for the lateral portion of the upper lateral incisors. The dual origin of each of the upper lateral incisors from *max'* and *premax* has relatively recently come to light from studies of individuals with cleft lip and from studies of subhuman primates [26, 27]. As further described below, patterns of incisor involvement provide important clues regarding clefting pathogenesis. Recent attention has also been paid to the origin and early development of the human nasal septum, with Steding and Jian [28], describing it as being derived from tissues located medial to the primary choanae. As shown in Fig. (**1.14a**), the nasal septum primordium has bilateral components that bound the medial borders of the primary nasal choanae. This relationship is also evident in Fig. (**1.16a**), which shows an 8 week-old fetus, and in which the primary nasal choanae have elongated antero-posteriorly. Both images illustrate the continuity between the developing nasal septum and the *premax*. Indeed, the nasal septum might be considered a derivative of a deep/posterior portion of the *premax* and/or *mnp* tissue.

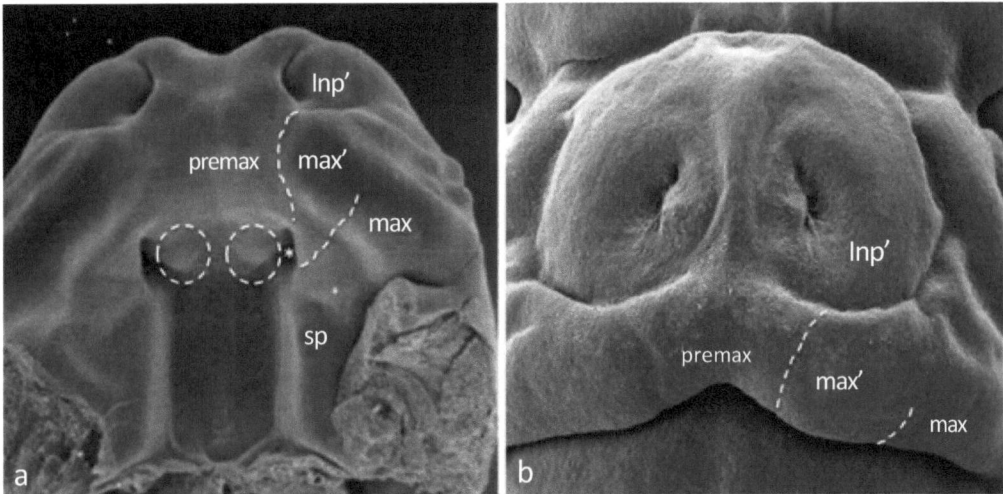

Fig. (**1.14**). Oral cavity and frontal views of a mouse embryo (a) and a slightly more advanced (46 day) human embryo (b), respectively, illustrate that while distinction between the facial growth centers is becoming less clear, the junction between premax and max' remains evident. Also apparent are bilateral components of the nasal septum (dashed circles) and their location medial to the primary choanae (*). sp = secondary palate.

The 8th week marks the end of the embryonic period. Fig. (**1.15**) shows that by this time, the discrete facial growth centers have become quite indistinguishable and that the eyelids have yet to form. Despite the relatively wide interocular distance and flattened midface, the facial appearance is distinctively human.

The beginning of the fetal period is marked by palatal fusion (Fig. **1.16**). This is preceded, in the 8th week, by a change in orientation/remodeling of the secondary palatal shelves such that they become positioned above the tongue instead of lateral to it. As previously shown (Figs. **1.12b**, **1.14a**), the secondary palatal shelves are bilateral medial extensions of the *max* growth centers. The definitive hard palate also has a small anterior component termed the primary palate that is of *premax* origin. While *max'* may also contribute to the anterior hard palate (esp. that portion associated with the distal segment of the upper lateral incisor), any such contribution has yet to be determined experimentally. The secondary palatal shelves begin their midline union at one third to one half of the distance from their anterior-most points (Fig. **1.16c**), with fusion proceeding both anteriorly (rostrally) and posteriorly. They also unite with the primary palate and with the nasal septum; union being complete by the end of the 9th week. The mechanisms involved in palatal closure and clefting have been the subject of extensive research [2]. Failure of the fusion process, itself, (*i.e.* the process of epithelial breakdown accompanied by convergence of the bilateral mesenchymal tissues), with insult occurring close to the time of normal secondary palatal closure can be the proximate cause of palatal clefting. Additionally, research has shown that in many (if not most) cases the proximate cause of typical palatal clefts is reduction in the size of the palatal shelves resulting from insult early in the genesis of the *max* center [29]. Abnormally increased distance between the palatal shelves resulting from excessive midfacial and forebrain width can also be the basis for some palatal clefts; esp. those associated with frontonasal dysplasia [30]; also see (Fig. **1.18**).

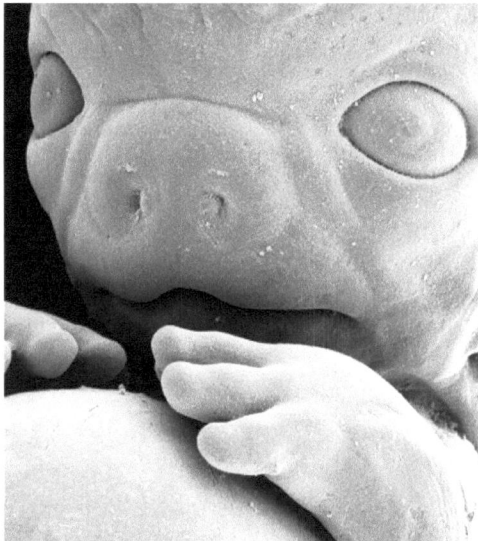

Fig. (1.15). By the mid-8th week, the facial features are distinctively human. At this time the eyelids have not yet formed; the nostrils are occluded by epithelial plugs; the ears remain low with respect to the lower jaw; and the fingers have formed.

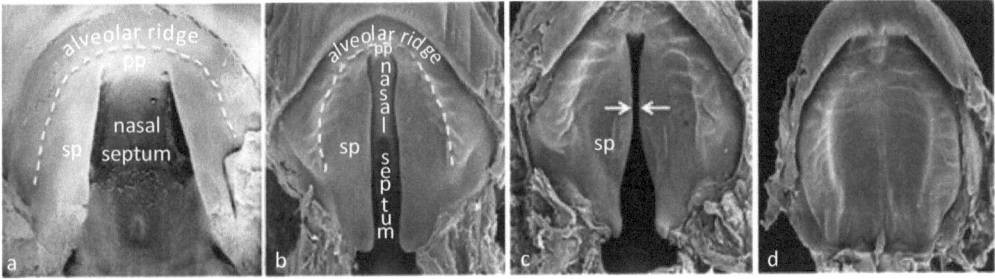

Fig. (1.16). The closing human palate is shown in human embryos at the end of the embryonic period (a; 55 days) and in the 9th week, which is the beginning of the fetal period (b-d). sp = secondary palatal shelf; pp = primary palate; arrows indicate approximate first site of secondary palatal fusion.

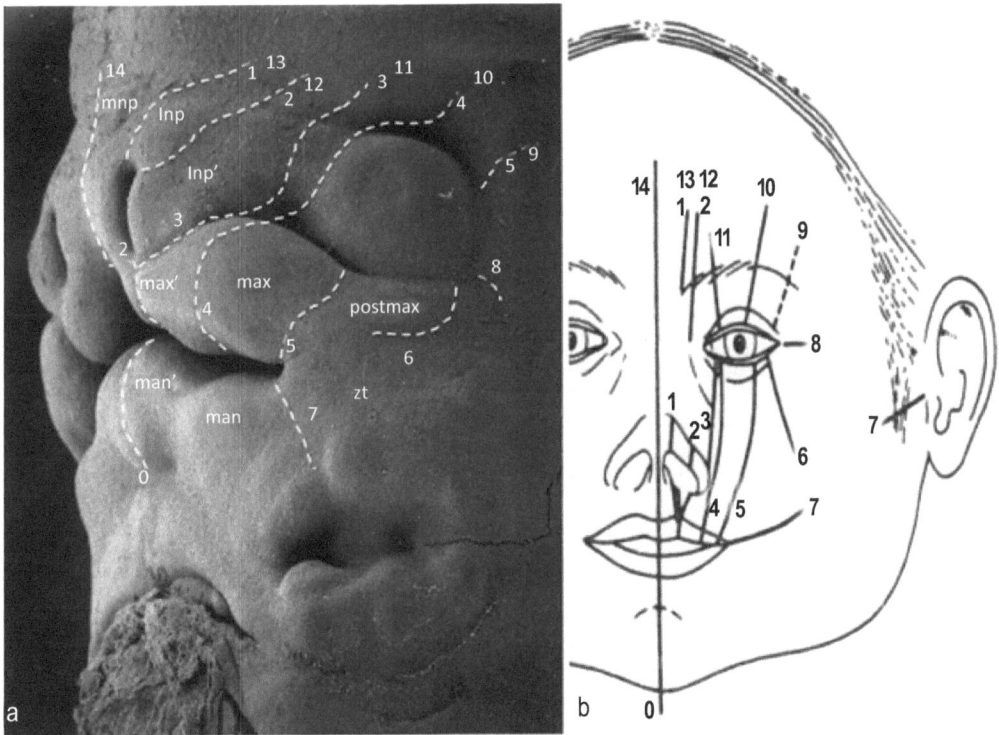

Fig. (1.17). Furrows between facial growth centers, most of which remain visible in the 7 week old human embryo shown in (a) correspond to facial clefting sites as described by Tessier (b; from Tessier [45]), and reflect a segmental developmental pattern.

EMBRYOGENESIS OF ORO-FACIAL CLEFTS

Oro-facial clefting sites are typically present at growth center junctions. This is readily appreciated in comparing the craniofacial clefting scheme developed by Tessier [1] to embryonic facial contours. While the genesis of the Tessier clefts will be discussed in further detail below, Fig. (**1.17**) provides a broad overview, with the surface location of each of the numbered clefts (including corresponding north- and south-bound clefts) related to the junctions of the oro-facial growth centers, most of which remain evident in the early 7th week human embryo shown. Overall, the pattern of clefts is indicative of a segmental origin for the growth center tissues. Indeed, it is likely that the *mnp, lnp, lnp', max', max, postmax* and the collective reminder of the first arch-associated growth centers *(zt, man, man')* represent separate rostro-caudally positioned streams or aggregates of neural crest cells; streams that are associated with specific neuronal segments. Also likely, and as reflected by the correspondence of the north- and south-bound clefts that are associated with the eye (3,11; 4,10; 5,9) is that acute teratogenic insult leading to these clefts occurs very early; at least prior to the time that the developing eye would interrupt the formation or positioning of the involved cellular aggregates (see Fig. **1.6**). Also possible is that molecular/genetic abnormalities specific to the individual facial and/or neuronal segments could be the basis for co-occurring north- and south-bound clefts.

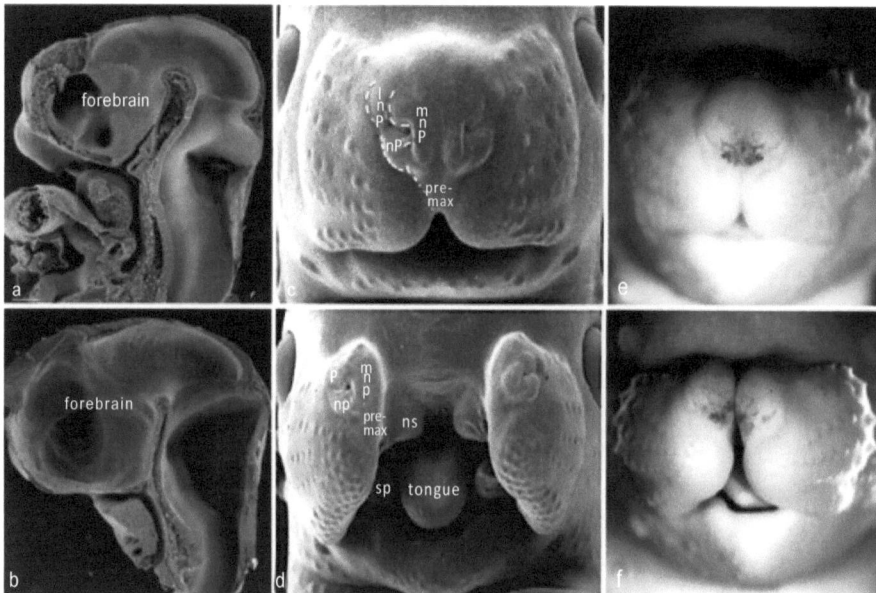

Fig. (1.18). Scanning electron micrographs (a-d) and light micrographs (e, f) of prenatal mice illustrate normal brain (a; mid-sagittal view) and facial (c, e) morphology, as compared to the brain and median facial defects induced by early teratogen exposure (b, d, f). The embryos shown in (b, d) were acutely exposed to methotrexate with brain distension resulting within hours of treatment, and with subsequent severe median facial clefts. The fetus shown in (f) that has a somewhat milder median facial cleft was acutely exposed to alcohol at a time corresponding approximately to the 22nd day of human development. Notable in the affected individuals is that all of the midfacial growth center-derived components of the nose and upper lip are present; that the mnp, premax, lnp, and lnp' of the mice shown in c-f can be identified; and that the bilateral components of the nasal septum (ns) and secondary palate (sp) remain separate in (d). Also notable is that by fetal stages, the mnp-derived nasal tip is becoming pigmented, with pigmentation being present in both the normal (e) and abnormal (f) mouse fetus.

Tessier's midline clefts (#0 and 14) of the midface are typically accompanied by hyperteleorbitism and a median frontal encephalocele. This type of cleft is, in fact, median craniofacial dysraphism, a defect that is commonly classified as frontonasal dysplasia. It involves a variable degree of abnormal midline separation between the combined *mnp* and *premax* centers on the right and left, as well as of the growth centers that will form the nasal septum and secondary palatal shelves. Although a midline cleft exists, all of the elements of the nose and upper lip are present and may be small, but are proportionally relatively normal. Differing degrees of severity of this type of cleft are shown in fetal mice in Fig. (**1.18**); the more severe defect shown in (b, d) resulting from maternal treatment with the antimetabolite, methotrexate, at a time corresponding to the 4th week of human gestation [30]. This drug treatment resulted in abnormal distension of the developing forebrain; a primary pathogenic factor underlying the median facial cleft. Another teratogen known to cause a combination of forebrain expansion and median facial clefts in animal models is alcohol (ethanol), with the critical exposure period for this defect being approximately equivalent to day 22 in humans (Fig. **1.18f**) [31, 32]. Notable is that in human populations and in animal models, mutation of genes that are critical for the function of primary cilia or of genes that signal through pathways requiring primary ciliary function can yield this type of cleft [33, 34]. Indeed, median facial clefts are now considered pathognomonic of a grouping of syndromes termed ciliopathies. Among the genes of particular interest whose products require primary cilia for developmental signaling is sonic hedgehog (SHH). The proper expression of this gene and its downstream targets is required for median forebrain development during the time of neural plate formation and neural tube closure. Studies by Brugmann and co-workers [33, 34] have shown that in genetically engineered mice excessive SHH activity, which can result from truncating primary cilia, can cause midfacial clefts. In this model, over-proliferation of neural crest cells was described as the primary basis for the defect.

In addition to midline clefts of the midface, the distal growth centers of the 1st pharyngeal arch (*man'*) may remain separate, the resulting defect being a median cleft of the lower jaw as shown in a mouse fetus in Fig. (**1.19**). In this individual, the malformation was subsequent to maternal treatment with retinoic acid at a time corresponding to the middle of the human 4th week of development; a time when a deep median furrow is normally present in the midline between the bilateral 1st pharyngeal arches [review Fig. (**1.8a**)].

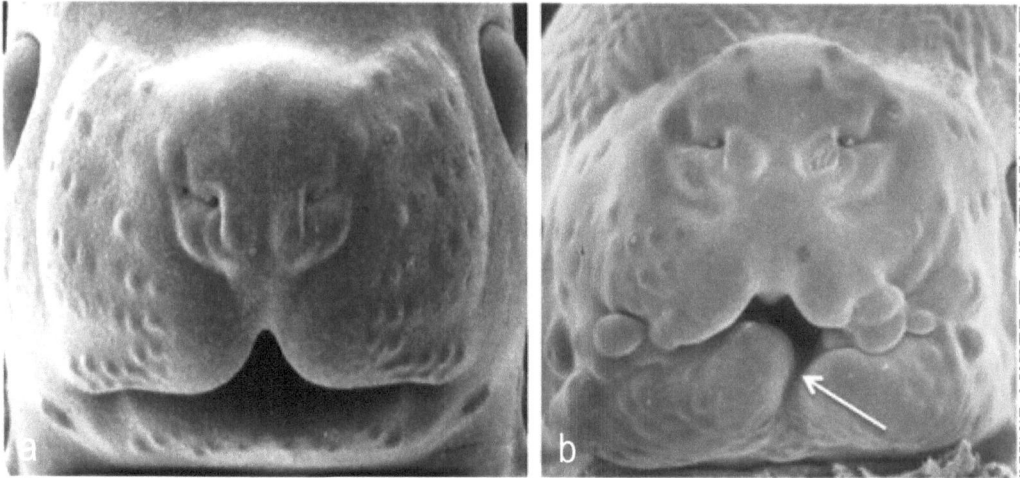

Fig. (1.19). As compared to the normal mouse fetus in (a), the retinoic acid-treated fetus in (b) has a median cleft of the lower jaw (arrow). Abnormal tissue tags are also present at the corners of the mouth of the latter.

Examination of mouse models is also helpful in appreciating the developmental basis for non-midline clefts. The abnormal mouse embryo shown in Fig. (**1.20b**) has defects consistent with Tessier's #1 and 13 clefts. Major deficiencies are apparent in the *mnp* components, while the *lnp* and the tissues that should come together to close the lip (*premax, lnp'*, and *max'*) appear to be of relatively normal size. However, with malpositioning of the *premax* segments, the lip is cleft bilaterally. Also notable are the presence of single forebrain hemisphere and failure of the anterior neuropore to close (a somewhat less severe presentation of this defect being frontal encephalocele).

Figs. (**1.21** and **1.22**) show the normal mouse fetus pictured above in Fig. (**1.18c**) for reference, along with fetuses having unilateral (Fig. **1.21b**), bilateral (Fig. **1.22b**), and incomplete (Fig. **1.22c**) upper lip clefts. In individuals with clefts, some of the growth centers are more readily defined than in normal animals at this stage of development. This is especially notable for *max'* which is clearly separate from *max* distally (Figs. **1.21b**, **1.22b**, **c**). Also, in a mouse fetus with bilateral cleft lip (Fig. **1.22b**), in one with incomplete clefts (Fig. **1.22c**), as well as in a child with bilateral cleft lip (Fig. **1.23b**) the facial surface of the *premax* appears excessively large. This is due to the failure of partial surface coverage by lateral tissues and a resulting totally unobscured *premax*.

As for the Tessier #1 cleft, in the type #2 and #3 clefts the upper lip defect is between the *premax* medially and the *lnp'* along with *max'* laterally. Deficiencies in any of these individual growth centers or in a combination of them may result in a gap that presents as a "typical" cleft lip. Highlighting the primary role of *premax* deficiency in some forms of cleft lip are experiments involving exposure of mouse embryos to SHH signaling antagonists [8, 35]. As shown in Fig. (**1.23**), defects ranging from apparently typical bilateral cleft lip, to bilateral cleft lip with a small *premax*, to median cleft lip with no *premax* can all result from exposure to this teratogen at times corresponding to the 4th week of human gestation. With the *premax* being the tissue in which the central incisors and mesial portion of the upper lateral incisors form, absence of these teeth is indicative of a primary pathogenic role for *premax* deficiency. Indeed, an individual with a cleft like that shown in Fig. (**1.23c**) would be expected to have no lateral incisors mesial to the cleft. This is the most common tooth pattern in individuals with "typical" cleft lip. An individual with a defect like that shown in Fig. (**1.23f**) would be expected to have neither central incisors nor the mesial component of the laterals. However, the portion of the lateral incisor distal to the cleft might be expected to be present in both cases. In the Tessier #2 cleft that is accompanied by its #12 north-bound counterpart, a defect in the *lnp'* and/or *lnp-* derived tissues that border the cleft occurs. In this cleft, the incisor sources (*premax* and *max'*) may not be deficient and lateral incisor components might be expected to be present on both sides of the cleft. In a Tessier #3 cleft that is accompanied by its #11 north-bound component a defect in *lnp'* and/or *max'* occurs. With *max'* involvement, absence of the portion of the lateral incisor distal to the cleft would be expected.

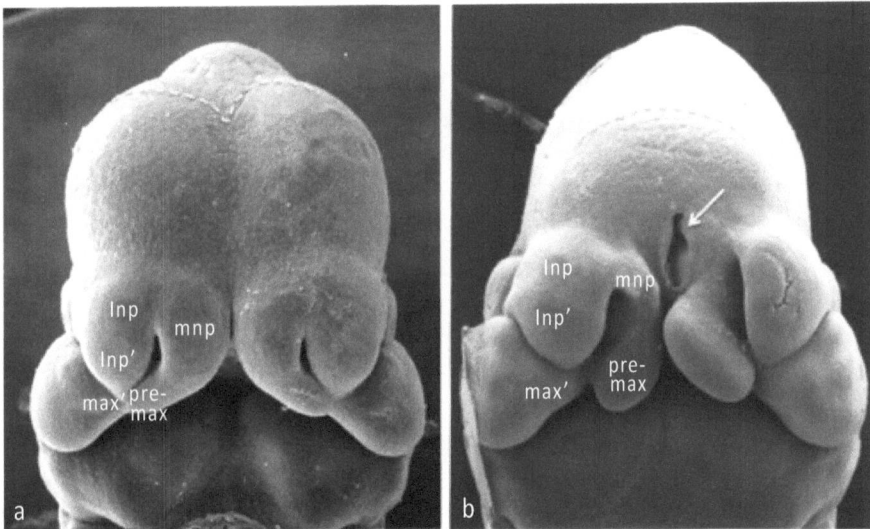

Fig. (1.20). Selective deficiency in the mnp of an abnormal mouse embryo (b), accompanied by malpositioning of the premax appear to be the basis for the combination of Tessier #1 and 13 clefts. The defects are somewhat asymmetric, with the mnp being virtually absent on the side with the less affected upper lip (embryo's left side), and present, but small, on the side with the wider gap in the upper lip. Arrow = open anterior neuropore; dashed lines indicate the contour of the telencephalon, a single cerebral hemisphere being present in the affected embryo.

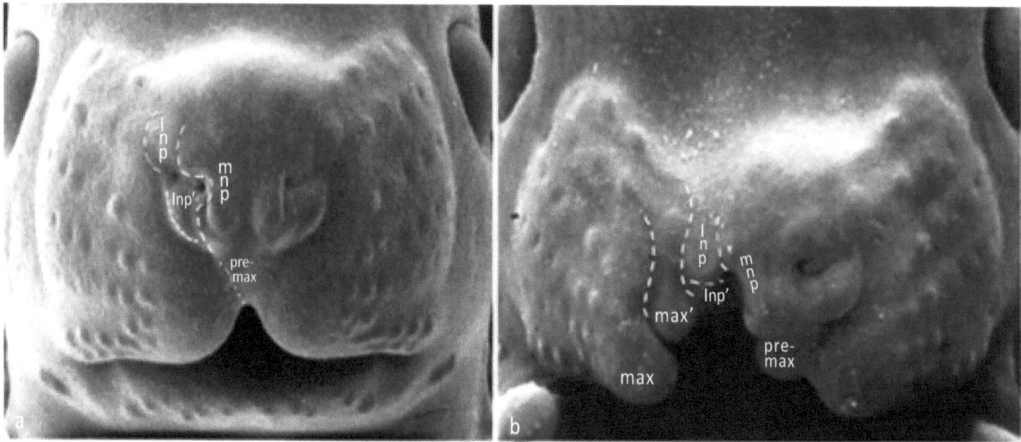

Fig. (1.21). Scanning electron micrographs illustrate a normal (a) and a unilateral cleft lip (b) in fetal mice. Notable in the latter is failure of union between the max' and lnp' with the premax. Also, noteworthy at the site of the cleft is the ready distinction between max' and max.

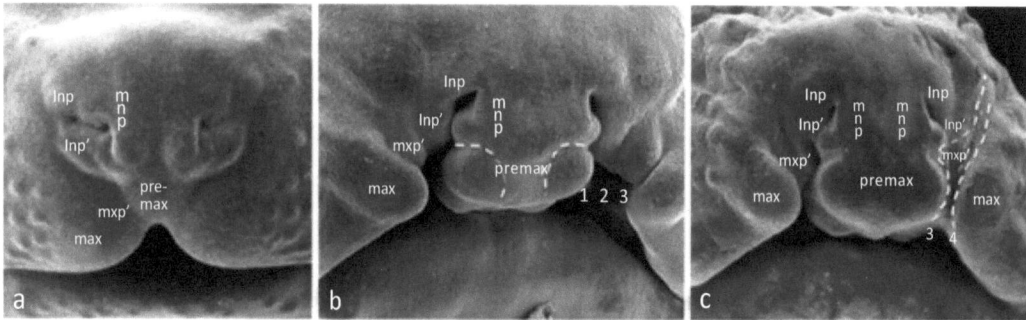

Fig. (1.22). Scanning electron micrographs of fetal mice illustrate a normal lip (a), along with bilateral (b) and incomplete (c) clefts of the lip that were induced with phenytoin at a time corresponding to the end of the 4th up to early in the 5th week of human development [36]. The dashed lines in (b) indicate the surface area of premax that is covered by lateral tissues in a normal upper lip. The dashed lines in (c) illustrate the position of the medial (distal) and lateral (proximal) borders of max'; the respective sites of an incomplete Tessier #3 cleft and of a #4 cleft.

Clefting at the lateral border of *max'*, at its junction with *max*, is consistent with Tessier #4 and #10 clefts, with the clefs resulting from deficiency in either or both of these growth centers and subsequent failure of their merging. The lip cleft is between the philtral ridge and the commissure of the mouth, with the cleft extending through the alveolar ridge between the upper lateral incisor and canine. This is in keeping with a *max'* origin of the upper lateral incisor and *max* origin of the canine. A mouse fetus with a Tessier #4 cleft is shown in Fig. (**1.22c**). The defect was caused by exposure to phenytoin at a time corresponding to the end of the 4th up to early in the 5th week of human development [36]; a time when the involved streams of *max'* and/or *max* neural crest cells remain unobstructed by the presence of the developing eyes (review Fig. **1.8**). Such an early time of insult to these cell populations appears to explain correspondence of the south-bound #4 cleft which is below the eye, and the #10, north-bound cleft above the eye.

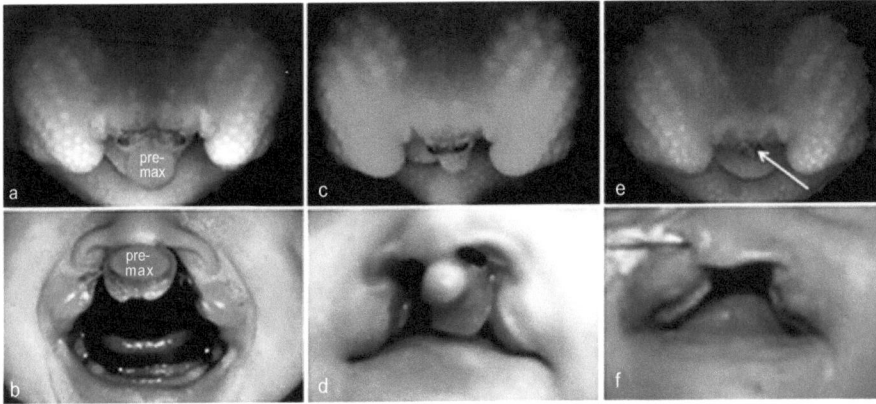

Fig. (1.23). Fetal mice treated with SHH antagonists at times corresponding to the human 4th week of gestation present with apparently typical bilateral cleft lip (a), bilateral cleft lip with a small premaxillary segment (c), and median cleft lip with no premaxillary segment (e). Respective human counterparts are shown in (b, d, f). Arrow in (e) indicates pigmented, mnp-derived tissue that remains in the absence of premax tissue. Modified from Lipinski *et al.* [8].

Tessier #5 and #9 clefts occur at the boundary between the *max* center (as defined herein) and the 1st pharyngeal arch (Fig. **1.24**). The #5 cleft extends from the outer corner of the mouth superficially, and deeply through the maxilla lateral to the maxillary sinus and through the alveolar ridge behind the canine in the premolar region. This cleft position is consistent with the *max* center giving rise to the medial/anterior part of the maxilla, and with the premise that all of the 1st pharyngeal arch derivatives are posterior/caudal to the #5 cleft. The origin of the posterior portion of the maxilla (that containing the premolars and molars) is tissue that is located between the position of the Tessier #5 and #6 clefts (Fig. **1.24b, c**). As opposed to the anterior part of the maxilla, the posterior part of the maxilla is 1st pharyngeal arch-derived.

In his classification scheme, Tessier groups clefts #6, 7 and 8 together as comprising the Treacher Collins-Franceschetti (TCS) syndrome. The deficiencies within this grouping involve the *postmax* and *zt* segment of the 1st pharyngeal arch (Fig. **1.24**). Recent studies have shown TCS to be causally associated with mutations in the TCOF1 gene. Mice that are haplo insufficient for this gene have increased neuroepithelial cell death and subsequently reduced numbers of neural crest cells migrating into the 1st and 2nd pharyngeal arches [37, 38]. Like genetic abnormalities, teratogen exposure can yield defects consistent with TCS. As shown in Fig. (**1.25**), mice exposed to retinoic acid for a brief time corresponding to early in the 4th week of human development present with reductions in the zygomaticotemporal region, including absence of the posterior aspect of the secondary palate. The pathology leading to these defects was shown to involve excessive cell death in the region of the developing trigeminal ganglion and placode, *i.e.* at the proximal margin of the 1st arch, which is the position of the #8 cleft [39].

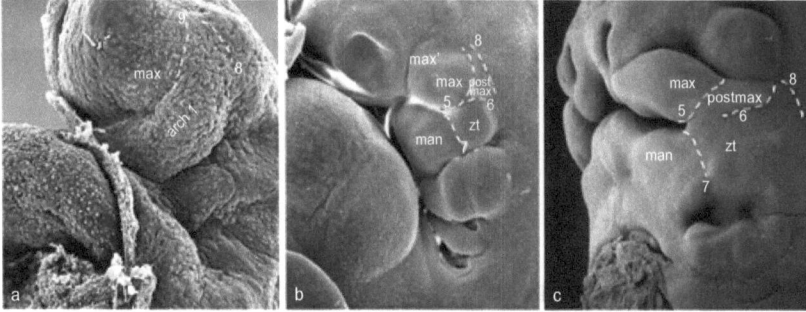

Fig. (1.24). Lateral views of human embryos at 25 (a), 37 (b) and 43 (c) days illustrate the position of Tessier #5-9 clefts. The #5 and 9 clefts are north- and south-bound counterparts that are at the junction of the max center and the 1st pharyngeal arch. The postmax is bounded by #5 and #6 clefts. The #7 cleft is at the junction between the zygomaticotemporal (zt) and mandibular (man) portions of the 1st arch. The #8 cleft is at the proximal border of the 1st arch, at the position of the trigeminal placode.

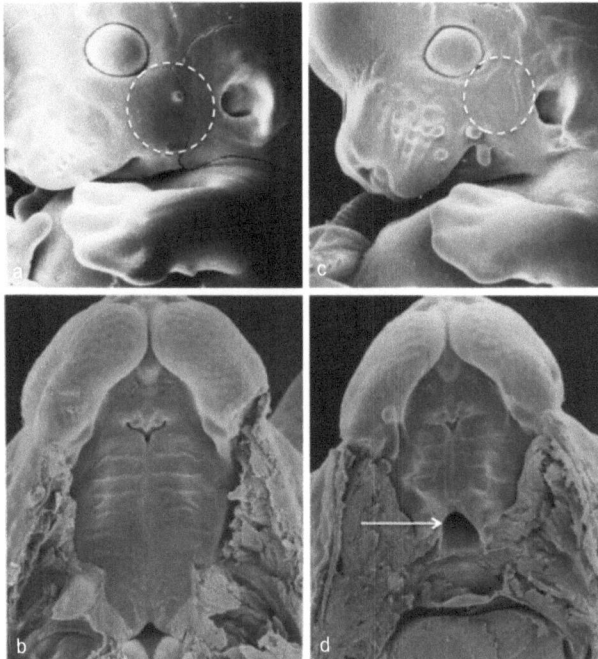

Fig. (1.25). Images of the face and secondary palate of a normal mouse fetus (a, b), and those of a fetus that had been exposed to retinoic acid at a time corresponding to early in the 4th week of human gestation (c, d) illustrate deficiency in the posterior maxillary and zygomaticotemporal region (dashed circles) and posterior portion of the secondary palate (arrow) in the latter. Modified from Sulik *et al.* [39].

EMBRYOGENESIS OF THE HOLOPROSENCEPHALY SPECTRUM

Defects within the holoprosencephaly (HPE) spectrum, which includes a broad range of co-occurring forebrain and midfacial malformations, have been reported in as many as 1:250 conceptuses and, with a high rate of prenatal demise in affected individuals, in approximately 1:8000 live births [11]. As determined in animal models, the developmental stages at which insult can lead to HPE are present during the middle of the 3rd through the beginning of the 4th week of human development [8, 29]. The tissues involved in the initial pathogenesis of HPE may include the prechordal plate, the adjacent endodermal and mesodermal cells, and/or the neuroepithelial cells of the ventro-medial forebrain (review Figs. **1.2** & **1.23**). A variety of both genetic and environmental factors (or a combination of them) can be causative. Of the known genetic causes, the most common are those that involve alterations in the sonic hedgehog (SHH) gene itself or genes encoding proteins that directly or indirectly regulate SHH expression or signaling [10, 40]. While the SHH signaling pathway is not the only one that when altered can yield HPE, it is notable that of the known environmental causes of HPE many are agents that directly or indirectly affect SHH-related cell signaling. Included are cholesterol biosynthesis inhibitors, cyclopamine, retinoic acid and alcohol. Noteworthy is that evidence for a gene/environment interaction involving alcohol lies in recent research showing that the birth defects that alcohol causes are more severe and occur with greater frequency in mice that are haploinsufficient for either SHH or a downstream gene (Gli2) than in normal, non-mutant mice [41].

That alcohol can cause HPE when administered at early stages of embryogenesis in non-mammalian model systems has been recognized for over 100 years [42]. Following up on this early research, Sulik and colleagues described the genesis of alcohol-induced HPE in mice, showing that a short window of prenatal alcohol exposure at times corresponding to the mid-3rd week of human gestation can yield a wide range of concurrent median forebrain and facial defects [8]. Fig. (**1.26**) shows dysmorphology that is apparent shortly after this early alcohol insult; dysmorphology that is characterized by abnormally close proximity of the olfactory placodes and subsequently of the nostrils. While the lateral aspects of the developing face, including the *lnps* and *max prominences* appear quite normal in these embryos, the *mnps* are too closely positioned, but still separate, in the more mildly affected embryo (Fig. **1.26e**), and are united to form a single central *mnp* in the more severely affected one (Fig. **1.26h**). The upper-midfacial deficiency co-occurs with loss of median forebrain tissue as is consistent with HPE (Fig. **1.26f, j**).

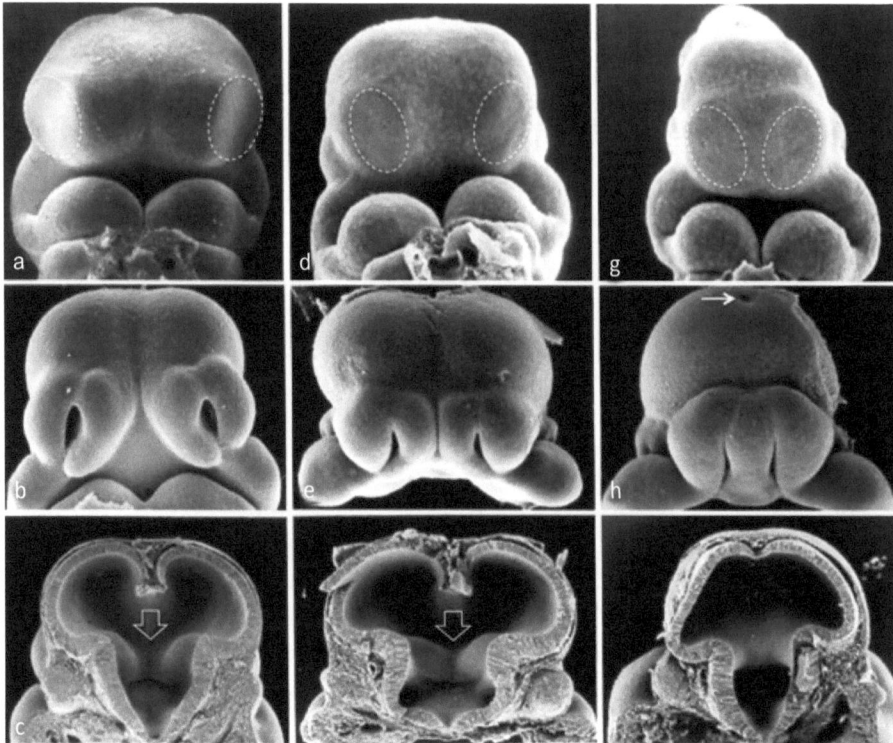

Fig. (1.26). Comparison of the developing face (a, b, d, e, g, h) and forebrain (c, f, i) of normal mouse embryos (a-c) and those showing varying degrees of holoprosencephaly (d-i) shows midline deficiency in the latter. At stages present in early 5th week humans, the olfactory placodes (dashed circles in a, d, g) of the abnormal embryos are too closely positioned. At stages present early in the 6th week of human development, this midline deficiency is reflected in too close proximity of the mnps as shown in (e) and (h) and in loss of median forebrain structures as shown in (f) and (i). Arrowhead in (h) = anterior neuropore abnormality; open arrows in (c) indicate median forebrain tissue that is deficient in (f) and absent in (i). Modified from Sulik and Johnson [43] and Sulik [43].

Shown in Fig. (**1.27**) is a wider range of alcohol-induced facial and brain defects as viewed in 3-D reconstructions of magnetic resonance images of mice at early fetal stages. Increasing severity of insult is reflected in increasingly close proximity of the nostrils and cerebral hemispheres to the point of nostril and cerebrum absence. In some animals the lower jaw is also affected, appearing too small (micrognathic) or even absent (agnathic) (Fig. **1.27g, i**). The faces of the affected animals are characterized by a long (from nose to mouth) upper lip. This is the result of abnormal medial convergence of the *max* prominences as can occur when the *premax* is too small or absent. Notably, a long upper lip with a deficient (*premax*-derived) philtrum is the phenotype that characterizes (full blown) fetal alcohol syndrome (FAS). Sulik and colleagues [44 - 46] suggest that full-blown FAS is, indeed, a form of HPE. While the brains of individuals with FAS do not typically present with single cerebral hemispheres (*i.e.* as holospheres), less severe midline forebrain defects, esp. corpus callosum deficiencies, occur [47]. In postnatal mice following human 3rd week equivalent alcohol exposure comparable corpus callosum abnormalities have been reported [48]. Of the fetuses shown in Fig. (**1.27**), the mildly affected individual in (c, d) has a phenotype that appears most consistent with FAS as it is currently clinically defined.

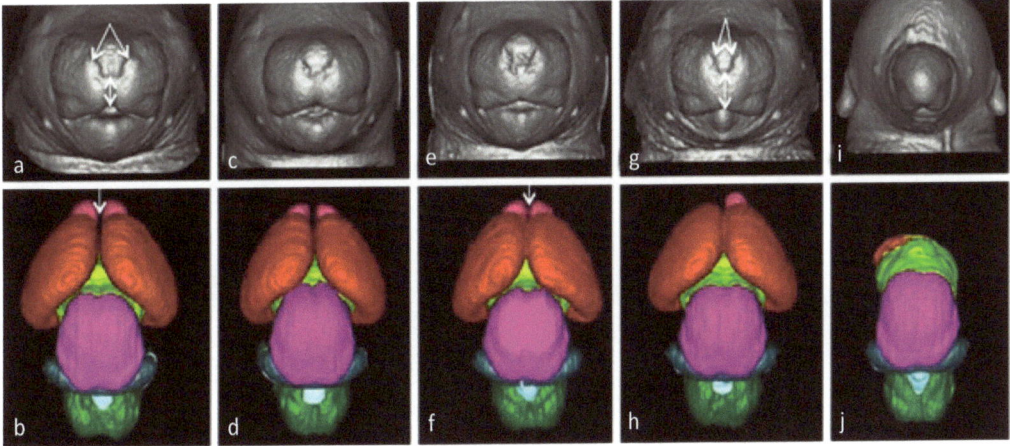

Fig. (1.27). 3-D reconstructed magnetic resonance images of the faces and brains of normal (a, b) and abnormal fetal mice that had been exposed to alcohol at a time corresponding to the mid-3rd week of human development (c-j) illustrate varying degrees of median facial and forebrain deficiency in the latter group. Arrows in (a) and (g) illustrate nostril proximity; double-headed arrows in (a) and (g) illustrate median upper lip length; arrows in (b) and (f) illustrate olfactory bulb (pink) and cerebral hemisphere (red) proximity; light green = diencephalon; magenta = mesencephalon; teal = cerebellum; dark green = remainder of rhombencephalon; blue = roof of 4th ventricle. Modified from Godin *et al* [13] & O'Leary-Moore *et al.* [48].

Both the alcohol-exposed severely affected mouse fetus shown in Fig. (**1.27i, j**) and that shown in Fig. (**1.28**) present with a rather extreme example of *max* prominence convergence as can occur in HPE. In these mice, not only is the *premax* absent, but the entirety of the *mnps* and *lnps* is also missing. This results in a lack of nasal structures and in formation of a snout that is surrounded by whisker follicles (structures that are exclusive to the *max* prominences). While the animal in Fig. (**1.27i, j**) has virtually no cerebrum, that in Fig. (**1.28**) has retained the lateral-most portions of its 2 cerebral hemispheres; these remaining parts of the cerebrum combining to form a holosphere. It is important to note that the commonly employed descriptor regarding the development of HPE is that it results from "inadequate or absent midline division of the forebrain into cerebral hemispheres"; a description that implies primary failure of an active forebrain cleavage process. This has created a misimpression since the basis for the defect is, instead, primary failure of the midline tissues of the forebrain to form.

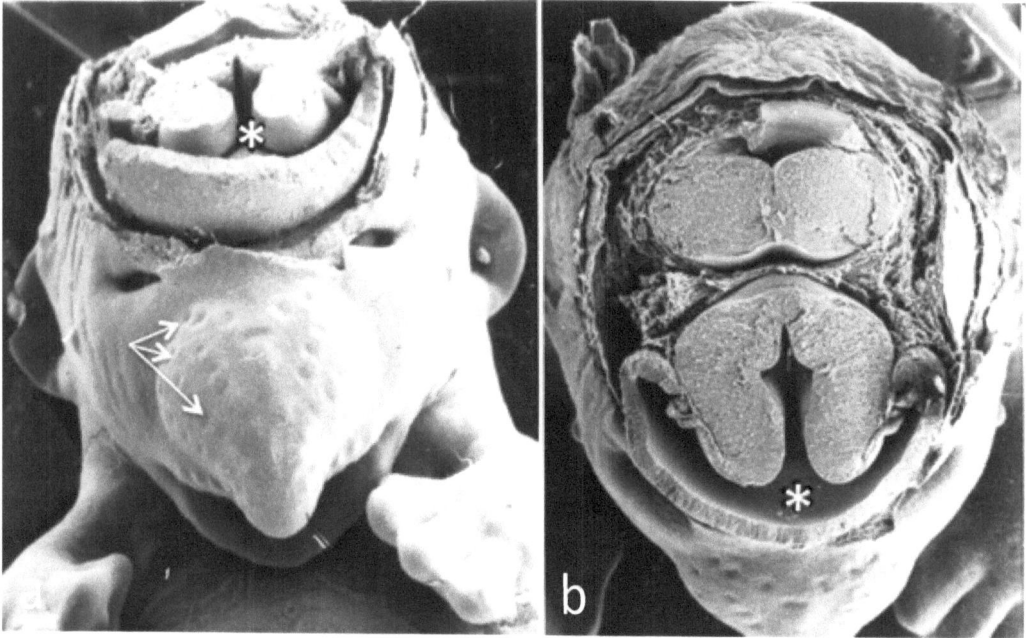

Fig. (1.28). A single (holoprosencephalic) cerebral hemisphere (*) is evident in a frontal (a) and dorsal view (b) of the transected head of an ochratoxin A-exposed fetal mouse. Arrows in (a) indicate whisker follicles on the snout. Modified from Wei and Sulik [49].

Figs. (**1.29** and **1.30**) are a composite of images illustrating many of the wide-ranging HPE-related facial phenotypes. Included are images of fetal mice with teratogen-induced defects and, for the milder end of the spectrum, images of children with corresponding abnormalities. The least pronounced defects shown are in a child with FAS (Fig. **1.29d**). Virtually the same upper midfacial phenotype, *i.e.* a long upper lip with philtral deficiency can occur in an individual who is agnathic as in Fig. (**1.29f**). Agnathia can also co-occur with more severe upper midfacial deficiencies as shown in Fig. (**1.30d**). The mandibular involvement and midline approximation of the external ears in agnathia/HPE (also termed otocephaly) appears to result from very early insult to the prechordal mesoderm.

The individuals in both Figs. (**1.29h**, and **j**) have a single nostril and are clearly hypoteloric, a phenotype termed cebocephaly. These individuals also have no philtrum and consequently have an upper lip vermillion without a cupid's bow; an upper lip in which *max* prominence tissues abnormally converge in the midline. The upper midfacial deficiency involves the *premax* and *mnps*, and median union of the olfactory placodes with preservation of the *lnps* from which the nose is formed. As shown in both a mouse fetus (Fig. **1.29i**) and a child (Fig. **1.29j**), this defect can co-occur with failure of the anterior neuropore to properly close;

presenting here as anencephaly. In some individuals that have *premax* agenesis the *max* prominence-derived tissues fail to converge in the midline, yielding a median cleft lip as in Fig. (**1.29k, l**) (see also Fig. (**1.23**)).

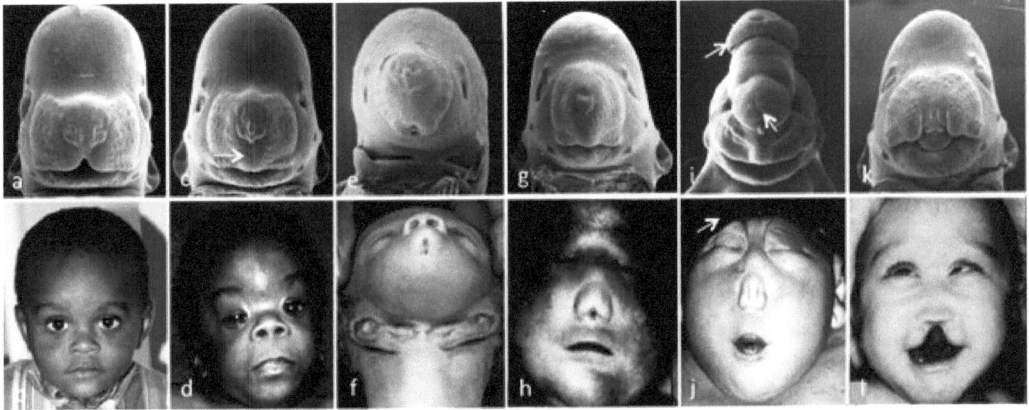

Fig. (1.29). As compared to normal (a, b) varying degrees of HPE are shown in fetal mice (c, e, g, I, k) and in children (d, f, h, j, l). Notable in the HPE group are hypoteleorism and philtral deficiency. This phenotype may be accompanied by anencephaly (arrows in i and j) and by micro- or agnathia, the latter of which presents as otocephaly (e, f).

Fig. (**1.30a**) shows an embryo that has features consistent with ethmocephaly, *i.e.* hypoteleorbitism with a proboscis between the eyes. A proboscis forms from the midline union of *lnp* tissues in the absence of *mnps*. Accompanying the abnormal brain development in HPE, the eyes may be positioned too far ventrally; a condition that in some cases can result in the proboscis being located above the eyes. This embryo also presents with very deficient *man* prominences, while the *max* prominences appear relatively more normal. As development proceeds this presentation is expected to yield micro- or agnathia.

When the midfacial deficiencies extend laterally enough to also involve the entire *lnps*, no proboscis forms, and instead the tissue between the closely positioned eyes is entirely *max* prominence-derived. In the mouse this tissue forms a whisker follicle-covered snout as previously described for the fetus in Fig. (**1.28**) and as also shown in Fig. (**1.30b, c, d**). Also evident in the latter figure is that the progressively greater tissue loss yields eyes that are united in the midline, the resulting synophthalmic structure being comprised of varying amounts of the more lateral components of both eyes. In these individuals, while the orbit might be considered cyclopic, the eyes should not as this wrongly implies that only one central eye was initially programmed to form from the forebrain tissue.

The loss of forebrain and facial tissue may be so extreme as to present as aprosencephaly. Shown in Fig. (**1.30e**), as compared to a normal fetus, no tissue is present beyond the level of the midbrain. Preservation of the midbrain allows the neural crest that populates the *max* prominences to form, while loss of more rostral tissues likely includes the prechordal mesoderm of the 1st pharyngeal arch and resultant lower jaw deficiency. It is rather remarkable and also troublesome to realize that in the absence of facial and forebrain tissue, the remainder of the body can develop quite normally to yield a term fetus.

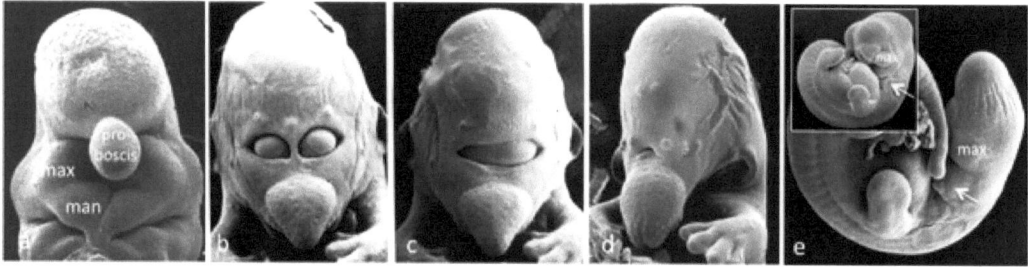

Fig. (1.30). Images of mouse embryos and fetuses illustrate facial features at the severe end of the HPE spectrum. The embryo in (a) presents with a proboscis, a structure that is derived from the *lnps*, and with deficient/abnormal *man* prominences (compare to Fig. (**1.20a**), which shows a comparably-staged normal embryo). The fetuses in (b-d) show increasingly close proximity (including median union) of the eyes and the presence of a whisker-follicle covered, *max* prominence-derived snout. The fetus in (d) is also agnathic. The aprosencephalic embryo in (e) is lacking facial tissue rostral to the *max* prominences and also has no forebrain. Arrows in (e) point to the 2nd pharyngeal arch in the abnormal embryo as well as in the comparably staged normal embryo shown in the inset. Modified, in part, from Wei and Sulik [49].

SUMMARY

Recognizing how incredibly complex and amazing normal embryogenesis is, it is not surprising that the process can be perturbed at countless steps along the way and in a multitude of manners. As detailed herein, many of the major malformations involving the face and brain, including those in the HPE spectrum, result from insult occurring in the 3rd through 4th weeks of prenatal development. This is a time when pregnancy typically remains unrecognized. Regarding HPE, it is clear that the wide-ranging phenotypes can result from both genetic and environmental causes or a combination of them. While defects at the severe end of the spectrum are readily identified pre- and postnatally, it is likely that the mildest forms frequently remain undetected and unclassified or misclassified.

Regarding typical and uncommon facial clefts, Tessier comments in his classic 1976 paper [1] that his classification scheme was developed based on personal clinical examination and surgical dissections; that is was theoretical and not dependent upon embryologic definition. As described herein, the morphology of human embryos and that of comparably staged experimental animals coupled with basic research results provide the basis for understanding the location of Tessier's well-defined clefting sites, showing that, indeed, they are embryologically-based. That it has taken so long to solidly reach this conclusion is undoubtedly the result of the common failure to recognize the presence and role of some of the key growth centers for oro-facial genesis. In particular, *lnp'* and *max'* have been overlooked, and the contribution and origin of the *max* center/prominence has been misunderstood. Identification of the presence and location of each of the growth centers allows the rostro-caudal segmental pattern of the oro-facies to be appreciated. This segmental pattern is established early in the embryonic period, is mirrored in Tessier's clefting sites, and provides a basis for understanding the concurrence of north- and south-bound clefts. Based on observational and experimental findings, the vast majority of oro-facial clefts appear to result from genetic and/or teratogenic insult occurring during the embryonic period, with the most likely proximate cause of clefting being failure of the normal growth and development of single or adjacent oro-facial growth centers.

CONFLICT OF INTEREST

The author (editor) declares no conflict of interest, financial or otherwise.

ACKNOWLEDGEMENTS

Research conducted in the author's laboratory has been generously supported by the US National Institute on Alcohol Abuse and Alcoholism, and has in part, been conducted as part of the Collaborative Initiative on Fetal Alcohol Syndrome *via* grant U01 AA021651.

REFERENCES

[1]   Tessier P. Anatomical classification facial, cranio-facial and latero-facial clefts. J Maxillofac Surg 1976; 4(2): 69-92.
[http://dx.doi.org/10.1016/S0301-0503(76)80013-6] [PMID: 820824]

[2]   Abbott BD. The etiology of cleft palate: a 50-year search for mechanistic and molecular understanding. Birth Defects Res B Dev Reprod Toxicol 2010; 89(4): 266-74.
[http://dx.doi.org/10.1002/bdrb.20252] [PMID: 20602452]

[3]   Bush JO, Jiang R. Palatogenesis: morphogenetic and molecular mechanisms of secondary palate development. Development 2012; 139(2): 231-43.
[http://dx.doi.org/10.1242/dev.067082] [PMID: 22186724]

[4]   Cordero DR, Brugmann S, Chu Y, Bajpai R, Jame M, Helms JA. Cranial neural crest cells on the move: their roles in craniofacial development. Am J Med Genet A 2011; 155A(2): 270-9.
[http://dx.doi.org/10.1002/ajmg.a.33702] [PMID: 21271641]

[5]   Dixon MJ, Marazita ML, Beaty TH, Murray JC. Cleft lip and palate: understanding genetic and environmental influences. Nat Rev Genet 2011; 12(3): 167-78.
[http://dx.doi.org/10.1038/nrg2933] [PMID: 21331089]

[6]   Gong SG. Cranial neural crest: migratory cell behavior and regulatory networks. Exp Cell Res 2014; 325(2): 90-5.
[http://dx.doi.org/10.1016/j.yexcr.2014.03.015] [PMID: 24680987]

[7]   Gritli-Linde A. The mouse as a developmental model for cleft lip and palate research. Front Oral Biol 2012; 16: 32-51.

[http://dx.doi.org/10.1159/000337523] [PMID: 22759668]

[8]   Lipinski RJ, Song C, Sulik KK, *et al.* Cleft lip and palate results from Hedgehog signaling antagonism in the mouse: Phenotypic characterization and clinical implications. Birth Defects Res A Clin Mol Teratol 2010; 88(4): 232-40.
[PMID: 20213699]

[9]   Minoux M, Rijli FM. Molecular mechanisms of cranial neural crest cell migration and patterning in craniofacial development. Development 2010; 137(16): 2605-21.
[http://dx.doi.org/10.1242/dev.040048] [PMID: 20663816]

[10]   Petryk A, Graf D, Marcucio R. Holoprosencephaly: signaling interactions between the brain and the face, the environment and the genes, and the phenotypic variability in animal models and humans. Wiley Interdiscip Rev Dev Biol 2015; 4(1): 17-32.
[http://dx.doi.org/10.1002/wdev.161] [PMID: 25339593]

[11]   Raam MS, Solomon BD, Muenke M. Holoprosencephaly: a guide to diagnosis and clinical management. Indian Pediatr 2011; 48(6): 457-66.
[http://dx.doi.org/10.1007/s13312-011-0078-x] [PMID: 21743112]

[12]   Twigg SR, Wilkie AO. New insights into craniofacial malformations. Hum Mol Genet 2015; 24(R1): R50-9.
[http://dx.doi.org/10.1093/hmg/ddv228] [PMID: 26085576]

[13]   Hinrichsen K. The early development of morphology and patterns of the face in the human embryo. Adv Anat Embryol Cell Biol 1985; 98: 1-79.
[http://dx.doi.org/10.1007/978-3-642-70754-4_1] [PMID: 4083112]

[14]   Sulik K, Dehart DB, Iangaki T, *et al.* Morphogenesis of the murine node and notochordal plate. Dev Dyn 1994; 201(3): 260-78.
[http://dx.doi.org/10.1002/aja.1002010309] [PMID: 7881129]

[15]   Basu B, Brueckner M. Cilia multifunctional organelles at the center of vertebrate left-right asymmetry. Curr Top Dev Biol 2008; 85: 151-74.
[http://dx.doi.org/10.1016/S0070-2153(08)00806-5] [PMID: 19147005]

[16]   Blum M, Schweickert A, Vick P, Wright CV, Danilchik MV. Symmetry breakage in the vertebrate embryo: when does it happen and how does it work? Dev Biol 2014; 393(1): 109-23.
[http://dx.doi.org/10.1016/j.ydbio.2014.06.014] [PMID: 24972089]

[17]   Komatsu Y, Mishina Y. Establishment of left-right asymmetry in vertebrate development: the node in mouse embryos. Cell Mol Life Sci 2013; 70(24): 4659-66.
[http://dx.doi.org/10.1007/s00018-013-1399-9] [PMID: 23771646]

[18]   Jacobson AG. Somitomeres: mesodermal segments of vertebrate embryos. Development 1988; 104 (Suppl.): 209-20.
[PMID: 3077109]

[19]   Meier S. Development of the chick embryo mesoblast. Formation of the embryonic axis and establishment of the metameric pattern. Dev Biol 1979; 73(1): 24-45.
[PMID: 527768]

[20]   Noden DM. The embryonic origins of avian cephalic and cervical muscles and associated connective tissues. Am J Anat 1983; 168(3): 257-76.
[http://dx.doi.org/10.1002/aja.1001680302] [PMID: 6650439]

[21]   Donkelaar HJ, Lammens M, Hori A, Eds. Clinical Neuroembryology. Heidelberg: Springer Verlag 2014.
[http://dx.doi.org/10.1007/978-3-642-54687-7]

[22]   Watson C, Paxinos G, Puelles L. The Mouse Nervous System. London: Academic Press 2012.

[23]   Smits-van Prooije AE, Vermeij-Keers C, Dubbeldam JA, Mentink MM, Poelmann RE. The formation

of mesoderm and mesectoderm in presomite rat embryos cultured *in vitro*, using WGA-Au as a marker. Anat Embryol (Berl) 1987; 176(1): 71-7.
[http://dx.doi.org/10.1007/BF00309754] [PMID: 3605652]

[24] Streeter GL. Developmental horizons in human embryos: age groups XV, XVI, XVII, and XVIII, being the third issue of a survey of the Carnegie Collection. Contrib Embryol 1948; 32: 133-203.

[25] Lee SH, Bédard O, Buchtová M, Fu K, Richman JM. A new origin for the maxillary jaw. Dev Biol 2004; 276(1): 207-24.
[http://dx.doi.org/10.1016/j.ydbio.2004.08.045] [PMID: 15531375]

[26] Hovorakova M1. Lesot H, Peterkova R, Peterka MJ. Origin of the deciduous upper lateral incisor and its clinical aspects. Dent Res 2006; 85: 167-71.
[http://dx.doi.org/10.1177/154405910608500210]

[27] Wei X, Senders C, Owiti GO, *et al.* The origin and development of the upper lateral incisor and premaxilla in normal and cleft lip/palate monkeys induced with cyclophosphamide. Cleft Palate Craniofac J 2000; 37(6): 571-83.
[http://dx.doi.org/10.1597/1545-1569(2000)037<0571:TOADOT>2.0.CO;2] [PMID: 11108527]

[28] Steding G, Jian Y. The origin and early development of the nasal septum in human embryos. Ann Anat 2010; 192(2): 82-5.
[http://dx.doi.org/10.1016/j.aanat.2010.01.002] [PMID: 20149609]

[29] Heyne GW, Melberg CG, Doroodchi P, *et al.* Definition of critical periods for Hedgehog pathway antagonist-induced holoprosencephaly, cleft lip, and cleft palate. PLoS One 2015; 10(3): e0120517.
[http://dx.doi.org/10.1371/journal.pone.0120517] [PMID: 25793997]

[30] Darab DJ, Minkoff R, Sciote J, Sulik KK. Pathogenesis of median facial clefts in mice treated with methotrexate. Teratology 1987; 36(1): 77-86.
[http://dx.doi.org/10.1002/tera.1420360111] [PMID: 3672380]

[31] Godin EA, O'Leary-Moore SK, Khan AA, *et al.* Magnetic resonance microscopy defines ethanol-induced brain abnormalities in prenatal mice: effects of acute insult on gestational day 7. Alcohol Clin Exp Res 2010; 34(1): 98-111.
[http://dx.doi.org/10.1111/j.1530-0277.2009.01071.x] [PMID: 19860813]

[32] Kotch LE, Sulik KK. Experimental fetal alcohol syndrome: proposed pathogenic basis for a variety of associated facial and brain anomalies. Am J Med Genet 1992; 44(2): 168-76.
[http://dx.doi.org/10.1002/ajmg.1320440210] [PMID: 1456286]

[33] Brugmann SA, Allen NC, James AW, Mekonnen Z, Madan E, Helms JA. A primary cilia-dependent etiology for midline facial disorders. Hum Mol Genet 2010; 19(8): 1577-92. a
[http://dx.doi.org/10.1093/hmg/ddq030] [PMID: 20106874]

[34] Brugmann SA, Cordero DR, Helms JA. Craniofacial ciliopathies: A new classification for craniofacial disorders. Am J Med Genet A 2010; 152A(12): 2995-3006. b
[http://dx.doi.org/10.1002/ajmg.a.33727] [PMID: 21108387]

[35] Lipinski RJ, Holloway HT, O'Leary-Moore SK, *et al.* Characterization of subtle brain abnormalities in a mouse model of Hedgehog pathway antagonist-induced cleft lip and palate. PLoS One 2014; 9(7): e102603.
[http://dx.doi.org/10.1371/journal.pone.0102603] [PMID: 25047453]

[36] Sulik KK, Johnston MC, Ambrose LJ, Dorgan D. Phenytoin (dilantin)-induced cleft lip and palate in A/J mice: a scanning and transmission electron microscopic study. Anat Rec 1979; 195(2): 243-55.
[http://dx.doi.org/10.1002/ar.1091950201] [PMID: 507390]

[37] Dixon J, Brakebusch C, Fässler R, Dixon MJ. Increased levels of apoptosis in the prefusion neural folds underlie the craniofacial disorder, Treacher Collins syndrome. Hum Mol Genet 2000; 9(10): 1473-80.
[http://dx.doi.org/10.1093/hmg/9.10.1473] [PMID: 10888597]

[38] Dixon J, Jones NC, Sandell LL, *et al.* Tcof1/Treacle is required for neural crest cell formation and proliferation deficiencies that cause craniofacial abnormalities. Proc Natl Acad Sci USA 2006; 103(36): 13403-8.
[http://dx.doi.org/10.1073/pnas.0603730103] [PMID: 16938878]

[39] Sulik KK, Johnston MC, Smiley SJ, Speight HS, Jarvis BE. Mandibulofacial dysostosis (Treacher Collins syndrome): a new proposal for its pathogenesis. Am J Med Genet 1987; 27(2): 359-72.
[http://dx.doi.org/10.1002/ajmg.1320270214] [PMID: 3474899]

[40] Roessler E, Belloni E, Gaudenz K, *et al.* Mutations in the human Sonic Hedgehog gene cause holoprosencephaly. Nat Genet 1996; 14(3): 357-60.
[http://dx.doi.org/10.1038/ng1196-357] [PMID: 8896572]

[41] Kietzman HW, Everson JL, Sulik KK, Lipinski RJ. The teratogenic effects of prenatal ethanol exposure are exacerbated by Sonic Hedgehog or GLI2 haploinsufficiency in the mouse. PLoS One 2014; 9(2): e89448.
[http://dx.doi.org/10.1371/journal.pone.0089448] [PMID: 24586787]

[42] Stockard C. The influence of alcohol and other anaesthetics on embryonic development. Am J Anat 2910(10): 369-92.

[43] Sulik KK. Critical periods for alcohol teratogenesis in mice, with special reference to the gastrulation stage of embryogenesis. Ciba Found Symp 1984; 105: 124-41.
[PMID: 6563984]

[44] Sulik KK. Genesis of alcohol-induced craniofacial dysmorphism. Exp Biol Med (Maywood) 2005; 230(6): 366-75.
[http://dx.doi.org/10.1177/15353702-0323006-04] [PMID: 15956766]

[45] Sulik KK, Johnston MC. Embryonic origin of holoprosencephaly: interrelationship of the developing brain and face. Scan Electron Microsc 1982; (Pt 1): 309-22.
[PMID: 7167750]

[46] Sulik KK, Johnston MC. Sequence of developmental alterations following acute ethanol exposure in mice: craniofacial features of the fetal alcohol syndrome. Am J Anat 1983; 166(3): 257-69.
[http://dx.doi.org/10.1002/aja.1001660303] [PMID: 6846205]

[47] Riley EP, Mattson SN, Sowell ER, Jernigan TL, Sobel DF, Jones KL. Abnormalities of the corpus callosum in children prenatally exposed to alcohol. Alcohol Clin Exp Res 1995; 19(5): 1198-202.
[http://dx.doi.org/10.1111/j.1530-0277.1995.tb01600.x] [PMID: 8561290]

[48] O'Leary-Moore SK, Parnell SE, Lipinski RJ, Sulik KK. Magnetic resonance-based imaging in animal models of fetal alcohol spectrum disorder. Neuropsychol Rev 2011; 21(2): 167-85.
[http://dx.doi.org/10.1007/s11065-011-9164-z] [PMID: 21445552]

[49] Wei X, Sulik KK. Pathogenesis of craniofacial and body wall malformations induced by ochratoxin A in mice. Am J Med Genet 1993; 47: 862-71.
[http://dx.doi.org/10.1002/ajmg.1320470613]

CHAPTER 2

Concepts of Genetics

Lucimara Teixeira das Neves[*], **Gisele da Silva Dalben**[*] and **Marcia Ribeiro Gomide**[*]

Bauru School of Dentistry and Hospital for Rehabilitation of Craniofacial Anomalies, University of São Paulo, Brazil

Abstract: This chapter aims to explain the basic concepts of genetics for the dental professional. Knowledge on the definitions of types of malformations, as well as the basis and nomenclature of genetic terms, will be fundamental for the readers to allow a thorough understanding on the aspects presented in Chapters 4 to 9.

Keywords: Congenital abnormalities, Embryonic development, Fetal development, Genetic structures, Genetic processes.

The congenital anomalies may involve a single organ, part of an organ or a wider region, and occur in the embryonic and fetal period. These anomalies affect 3 to 5% of the world population. These disorders may be hereditary or not. They are usually characterized as hereditary when they present a probable known genetic component in their etiology, and may present a characteristic inheritance pattern or not, observable by evaluation of the family history. Depending on this pattern, the disorder may or may not be transmitted to the offspring, regardless of its manifestation or extent [1].

The congenital anomalies are classified as:

- Developmental field anomalies: these affect part of the embryo in which the development occurs. They alter the differentiation of totipotent cells into specialized cells, causing anomalies in structures at the same site or stage of embryonic development. When caused by a teratogenic agent, the earlier the

[*] **Corresponding author Lucimara Teixeira das Neves:** Bauru School of Dentistry and Hospital for Rehabilitation of Craniofacial Anomalies, University of São Paulo, Bauru, Brazil; Tel/Fax: +55 14 3235-8000; E-mail: lucimaraneves@fob.usp.br
[*] **Gisele da Silva Dalben:** Hospital for Rehabilitation of Craniofacial Anomalies, University of São Paulo, Bauru, Brazil; Tel/Fax: +55 14 3235-8000; E-mail: gsdalben@usp.br
[*] **Marcia Ribeiro Gomide:** Hospital for Rehabilitation of Craniofacial Anomalies, University of São Paulo, Bauru, Brazil; Tel/Fax: +55 14 3235-8000; E-mail: marcinha@usp.br

action of the agent, the greater will be the damage. Example: Opitz G/BBB syndrome.

- Sequences: multiple anomalies in different structures derived from a single primary defect, known or assumed, or even a mechanical factor that triggers a cascade of secondary events determining abnormal characteristics. Example: Robin sequence (micrognathia – glossoptosis – cleft palate) [2, 3].
- Syndromes: patterns of multiple anomalies with pathogenic interrelation that do not represent developmental field anomalies or sequences. Some syndromes present known etiology, such as monogenic syndromes and chromosomopathies. Especially in cases of monogenic syndromes, in many cases there is an identifiable pattern of inheritance in the family; however, they may present variable expressivity and reduced penetrance. One such example is the van der Woude syndrome, which presents high penetrance and variable expressivity, exhibiting characteristic of monogenic disease caused by mutation in the *IRF6* gene [4 - 6].
- Associations: multiple anomalies occurring in higher frequency than expected by casualty, which cannot be classified as developmental field anomaly, sequence or syndrome. They have tendency to appear in combination, yet without family recurrence (only 2% of cases). The signs of associations may vary between children. If an association exhibits an identifiable inheritance pattern, it is then considered a syndrome. Some examples are: coloboma, heart disease, choanal atresia, delayed growth and development, genital alterations, ear anomalies (CHARGE association).
- Isolated defects: these affect only one body system and represent two thirds of all congenital anomalies.

Regarding the magnitude of anomalies, major anomalies are defined as alterations causing important functional impairment, such as cleft lip and palate and heart diseases. Conversely, the minor anomalies cause only esthetic disorders, such as preauricular tags. However, minor anomalies may indicate the presence of more severe disorders or even syndromes. Any child with more than three minor anomalies should be investigated in detail to rule out the possibility of syndromes [7].

There are several pathogenetic mechanisms of congenital anomalies, which include:

- Anomalies of organogenesis: affect an organ, part of an organ or a wider body region. These malformations involve an intrinsically abnormal embryonic primordium (example: cleft lip and palate), thus the term *congenital malformation* is redundant. Disruptions refer to an alteration in normal development due to an extrinsic factor, especially during the first trimester of pregnancy; and the earlier the action of the disruptive agent, the more severe the anomaly (example: amniotic bands) (Figs. **2.1, 2.2** and **2.3**).

- Anomalies of fetal life development: mechanical forces that affect the configuration of body structures that could potentially present normal development. These affect mainly the bones, cartilages and joints, and are called deformations. Example: isolated craniosynostosis caused by abnormal position in the womb or narrow maternal pelvis.
- Anomalies of histogenesis: structural alterations with clinical evidences, caused by abnormal organization or function of a specific tissue. They may not be visible at birth, worsening and allowing diagnosis over time. Example: skeletal dysplasia.

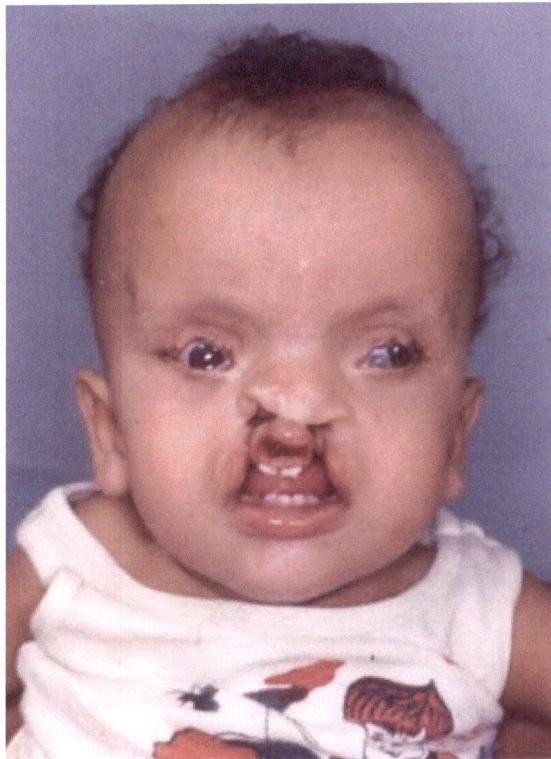

Fig. (2.1). Individual with amniotic band syndrome – facial aspect.

Fetal movement is fundamental for the adequate formation. Its restriction causes deformation (example: lack of amniotic fluid – oligohydramnios). The occurrence of polyhydramnios may also indicate the presence of fetal anomaly (the child may not be swallowing the amniotic fluid).

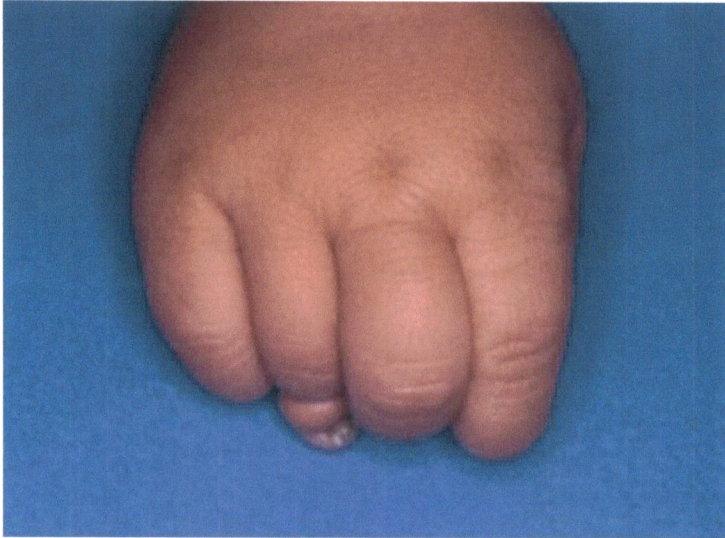

Fig. (2.2). Individual with amniotic band syndrome – hand.

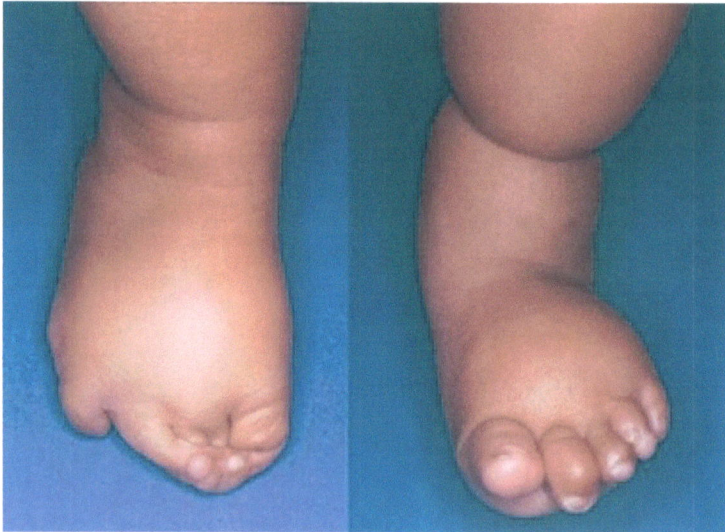

Fig. (2.3). Individual with amniotic band syndrome – feet.

DIAGNOSIS IN DYSMORPHOLOGY

The diagnosis in dysmorphology aims to establish the clinical diagnosis and possibly the etiologic factor, guiding the treatment (when possible) and allowing genetic counseling. For that purpose, the following steps are necessary:

A. anamnesis/genogram for description of anomalies and graphic representation of the family context;

B. definition of major and minor signs, with synthesis of clinical findings for analysis and identification of the probable etiology when possible;

C. utilization of diagnostic resources (literature, computer software, and laboratory cytogenetic and molecular laboratories when available);

D. re-evaluation for confirmation of initial clinical findings and analysis of new characteristics that may appear

E. diagnostic hypothesis or conclusion

F. genetic counseling

POPULATION GENETICS

Human species is differentiated by ethnicities and, secondly, by variations in the DNA sequence. This field of study aims to analyze the events occurring in isolated populations.

Hardy [8] and Weinberg [9], independent researchers, proposed the same theory at different places. Their theory would be valid for closed populations with ideal reproduction conditions. In these populations, the proportion of heterozygous individuals does not change and the frequencies of genes remain constant.

In the Brazilian population, this balance may be affected by preferential marriage (class, affinity, consanguinity) and migration flow (mixed pool of genes). Migrations may alter the genetic characteristics and habits of the population, both at arrival and departure. These factors raise the need of epidemiological studies also taking the environment into account. One example of such studies is the Latin American Collaborative Study of Congenital Malformations (ECLAMC).

The compilation of collective epidemiological data is complex, since it relies on the voluntary compliance of professionals involved in the attention and adequate filling of birth certificates. The epidemiological surveillance programs and case-control studies are important to identify possible etiologic factors related to the occurrence of congenital anomalies.

The epidemiological evaluation of complex craniofacial malformations is further complicated by the relatively low prevalence of each type of malformation and the high phenotypical variability.

BASIC CONCEPTS OF GENETICS

The genetic information in humans, the human genome, is composed of nuclear DNA (99%) and mitochondrial DNA (1%) [10].

Nucleotides are the primary molecules composing the DNA, which are biochemically composed of a phosphate group, a sugar group (deoxyribose) and nitrogenous bases. These bases belong to two different groups, namely the purines, represented by adenine and guanine; and pyrimidines, represented by cytosine and thymine. From the standpoint of three-dimensional characteristic, the DNA molecule presents as a double helix in which the phosphate and sugar group constitute the invariable region, *i.e.* the molecule framework, and the bases are the variable regions, maintained inside the DNA structure by hydrogen bonds. This pairing between nitrogenous bases occurs by complementarity and they remain joined due to the hydrogen bonds, with two bonds uniting adenine and thymine and three bonds joining cytosine and guanine, as well as due to the hydrophobic characteristics of the DNA molecule. The nitrogenous bases in the nucleotide structure represent the genetic code of each individual.

The DNA molecule is a long structure compacted in chromosomes inside the cell nucleus. Chromosome is a Greek-derived word (kroma=shade, soma=body), being defined as a spiral filament of chromatin, present inside the nucleus of all cells. This chromatin is composed of DNA molecule (deoxyribonucleic acid) associated with a group of different proteins. From an organizational standpoint, the chromosomes contain the genes, which are conceptually considered the DNA coding regions and ultimately allow the hereditary transmission of characteristics [11].

In their structural-morphological structure, each mitotic chromosome presents a constriction named centromere, which is considered a reference point that divides the chromosomes in two arms: p (from the French word petit = small), the short body; and q (from the French word queue= tail), the long arm. Chromosomes are described according to the pair number to which they belong, and the position of genes in the chromosome structure are defined according to the arm where they are located; *e.g.* 10q is the long arm of chromosome 10. To define the exact position of a gene in the chromosome, each arm is divided in numbered regions. For example, the etiology of Apert syndrome is related to the gene located at the region 10q26.

The collection of chromosomes in the nucleus of somatic cells in mankind is composed of 23 pairs of chromosomes. Among these, 22 pairs (numbered from 1 to 22) are similar in both genders, being called autosomal chromosomes; the other pair corresponds to the sexual chromosomes and present different morphologies between each other, defined as XX for females and XY for males. This typical collection of chromosomes may be analyzed by the karyotype, which is widely used as diagnostic means for detection of chromosomal anomalies, investigating numerical and structural alterations of chromosomes.

Another important aspect related to the chromosomes and their nomenclature concerns the definition of the inheritance pattern of a certain characteristic or disease, especially monogenic diseases. One example is the van der Woude syndrome, which is a disorder with autosomal dominant inheritance pattern, meaning that the mutation in the *IRF6* gene, the etiologic factor of this syndrome, is located in an autosomal chromosome and that the mutation in only one allele of the pair will determine the phenotypic expression of the syndrome in the individual presenting the variation.

CONFLICT OF INTEREST

The author (editor) declares no conflict of interest, financial or otherwise.

ACKNOWLEDGEMENTS

Declared none.

REFERENCES

[1]   Nussbaum RL, McInnes RR, Willard HF. Thompson & Thompson Genetics in Medicine. Philadelphia: Elsevier/Saunders 2007.

[2]   Côté A, Fanous A, Almajed A, Lacroix Y. Pierre Robin sequence: review of diagnostic and treatment challenges. Int J Pediatr Otorhinolaryngol 2015; 79(4): 451-64.
[http://dx.doi.org/10.1016/j.ijporl.2015.01.035] [PMID: 25704848]

[3]   Gangopadhyay N, Mendonca DA, Woo AS. Pierre robin sequence. Semin Plast Surg 2012; 26(2): 76-82.
[http://dx.doi.org/10.1055/s-0032-1320065] [PMID: 23633934]

[4]   Deshmukh PK, Deshmukh K, Mangalgi A, Patil S, Hugar D, Kodangal SF. Van der woude syndrome with short review of the literature. Case Rep Dent 2014; 2014: 871460.
[http://dx.doi.org/10.1155/2014/871460]

[5]   Drew SJ. Clefting syndromes. Atlas Oral Maxillofac Surg Clin North Am 2014; 22(2): 175-81.
[http://dx.doi.org/10.1016/j.cxom.2014.05.001] [PMID: 25171998]

[6]   Kaul B, Mahajan N, Gupta R, Kotwal B. The syndrome of pit of the lower lip and its association with cleft palate. Contemp Clin Dent 2014; 5(3): 383-5.
[http://dx.doi.org/10.4103/0976-237X.137961] [PMID: 25191078]

[7]   Monlleó IL, de Barros AG, Fontes MI, de Andrade AK. de M Brito G, do Nascimento DL, Gil-d--Silva-Lopes VL. Diagnostic implications of associated defects in patients with typical orofacial clefts. J Pediatr in press

[8]   Hardy GH. Mendelian proportions in a mixed population. Science 1908; 28(706): 49-50.
[http://dx.doi.org/10.1126/science.28.706.49] [PMID: 17779291]

[9]   Weinberg W. Über den Nachweis der Vererbung beim Menchen. Jahresh Ver Vaterl Naturkd Wurttemb 1908; 64: 368-82.

[10]   Griffiths AJ, Wessler SR, Lewontin RC, Carroll SB. Introduction to genetic analysis. Dallas: W. H. Freeman and Company 2007.

[11]   Robinson WN, Borges-Osório MR. Genética para Odontologia. Porto Alegre: Artemed 2006.

CHAPTER 3

Teratology and Teratogens

Lucimara Teixeira das Neves[*]

Bauru School of Dentistry and Hospital for Rehabilitation of Craniofacial Anomalies, University of São Paulo, Brazil

Abstract: This chapter presents the mechanisms of teratogenesis and depicts the main teratogens involved in disorders of craniofacial development. This knowledge will aid the understanding on aspects presented in Chapters 4 to 9.

Keywords: Teratology, Teratogenesis, Teratogens.

The term teratogenesis (terat=monster) refers to an interference during prenatal development, causing congenital anomalies. Teratology is the investigation of contribution of external factors potentially able to alter the intricate and complex prenatal development. Teratogens are the chemical, physical, biological agents and maternal disorders that may cause these congenital defects. These agents are also investigated as to the means through which they may adversely affect the intrauterine environment of the developing fetus. These factors may act by heterogeneous pathogenic mechanisms, inducing severe alterations with loss of the embryo or fetus, may cause morphological and functional anomalies (including growth) or even neurobehavioral disorders (learning and behavior disorders) [1].

The teratogens may act in isolation or associated with a genetic predisposition, consequently causing an anomaly, and this pattern of occurrence of congenital anomalies is called multifactorial etiology. For many pathologies that present this type of pattern, the weight of contribution of predisposing genetic factors and teratogens, also called environmental factors, are not yet clearly defined. One example of malformation with this characteristic is the non-syndromic (isolated) cleft lip and palate [2].

The mechanisms of action of teratogens usually present some selectivity as to the

---

[*] **Corresponding author Lucimara Teixeira das Neves:** Bauru School of Dentistry and Hospital for Rehabilitation of Craniofacial Anomalies, University of São Paulo, Bauru, Brazil; Tel/Fax: +55 14 3235-8000; E-mail: lucimaraneves@fob.usp.br

target and effect. Therefore, it is expected that characteristic patterns of anomalies may be associated with specific teratogens. However, the extent to which the individual may be affected by exposure to a certain teratogen is variable. This variability results in differences in clinical phenotypes, due to differences in the dose, period of prenatal development upon exposure, differences in individual susceptibility and interactions between environmental exposures to different agents.

For this reason, it would not be adequate to restrict the consideration only to the most severe end of the spectrum, in which a promptly recognizable pattern – a syndrome – appears frequently. Thus, a terminology that includes several outcomes should be used. The term "fetal effects" describes this variation more adequately and includes the milder end of the spectrum, usually not considered as a classical "syndromic" individual.

Apparently, teratogens do not seem to be effective in causing abnormalities in the first two weeks of development. However, their action at this early and fundamental stage may lead to embryo death. In the following stage, corresponding to the embryonic period (3rd to 8th week), there is greater susceptibility, constituting a critical period for the occurrence of malformations if the embryo is exposed to these agents [3].

It should be highlighted that the action of a teratogen causing abnormalities, as well as the severity of these abnormalities, depends basically on four aspects: timing of exposure, dose, specific pathogenic mechanism and genotype of the embryo and mother, which are related to characteristics of individual resistance to these agents [4].

TERATOGENS

Some of the best known teratogens related with craniofacial malformations and some of their effects are listed below [5]:

- Ethyl alcohol: fetal alcohol syndrome (alterations in the central nervous system, cardiovascular disorders, growth deficiency, short palpebral fissures, short nose, hypoplastic philtrum, hypoplastic maxilla, retrognathia during childhood, microcephaly, microphthalmia, micrognathia, thin upper lip; broad nasal base [6, 7];
- Vitamin A and derivatives: microcephaly, hydrocephaly, facial paralysis, facial asymmetry, hypoplastic middle facial third, metopic synostosis, microphthalmia, oculomotor palsy, cleft lip and palate, microtia, holoprosencephaly, femoral hypoplasia, craniosynostosis, syndactyly, abnormalities in the central nervous system, external ear, thymus, cardiovascular and genitourinary disorders;

- Folic acid antagonists: prenatal growth deficiency, hydrocephaly, intellectual disability, wide cranial sutures with delayed mineralization, cranial lacunae, abnormal cranial shape, craniosynostoses, anencephaly, spina bifida, hyperteleorbitism, micrognathia, cleft palate, absence or hypoplasia of digits, syndactyly, alterations in the central nervous system, ear, long bones and ribs;
- Anticoagulant (coumadin): warfarin syndrome, prenatal growth deficiency, delayed neuropsychomotor development (DNPMD), microcephaly, hydrocephaly, agenesis of the brain, occipital meningoencephalocele, agenesis of the corpus callosum, hearing impairment, hypoplastic middle facial third, nasal hypoplasia, mammary hypertelorism, anomalies of the central nervous system, midline, ocular and cardiovascular alterations;
- Hydantoin: prenatal growth deficiency, functional disorders of the central nervous system, craniofacial and limbs dimorphism, hypoplastic middle facial third, short nose, broad and low nasal bridge, epicanthal folds, mild hyperteleorbitism, ptosis, strabismus, marked cupid's bow, short neck, cleft lip and palate, cardiac and genitourinary alterations;
- Oxazolidinedione: microcephaly, characteristic facial aspect with flattened middle facial third, short nose, epicanthal folds, strabismus, myopia, meningomyelocele, cleft palate, scoliosis, cardiovascular, ear and genitourinary disorders;
- Valproic acid: trigonocephaly, narrow frontal diameter, hypoplastic middle facial third, short nose with wide nasal bridge, long and wide philtrum, micrognathia, cleft lip and palate, tracheomalacia, lumbosacral meningomyelocele, ear, genital, cardiac and limb disorders;
- Mercury: microcephaly, cerebral palsy, intellectual disability;
- Anti-cancer drugs: DNPMD, cleft palate, ocular, genitourinary and limb alterations;
- Antibiotics (streptomycin, kanamycin, aminoglycosides, chloroquine): hearing impairment;
- Virus (rubella, cytomegalovirus, herpes simplex, varicella zoster): ocular and cardiovascular alterations, hearing impairment, hepatosplenomegaly, DNPMD [8, 9];
- Bacteria (Treponema pallidum): DNPMD, ocular, dental and skeletal alterations;
- Diabetes mellitus: facial clefts, holoprosencephaly, cardiovascular, renal and neural tube alterations;
- Phenylketonuria: DNPMD, microcephaly, cardiac and vertebral defects, fetal death.

CONFLICT OF INTEREST

The author (editor) declares no conflict of interest, financial or otherwise.

ACKNOWLEDGEMENTS

Declared none.

REFERENCES

[1]   Toralles MB, Trindade BM, Fadul LC, Peixoto Junior CF, Santana MA, Alves C. A importância do Serviço de Informações sobre Agentes Teratogênicos, Bahia, Brasil, na prevenção de malformações congênitas: análise dos quatro primeiros anos de funcionamento. Cad Saude Publica 2009; 25(1): 105-10.
      [http://dx.doi.org/10.1590/S0102-311X2009000100011] [PMID: 19180292]

[2]   Freitas JA, das Neves LT, de Almeida AL, *et al.* Rehabilitative treatment of cleft lip and palate: experience of the Hospital for Rehabilitation of Craniofacial Anomalies/USP (HRAC/USP)--Part 1: overall aspects. J Appl Oral Sci 2012; 20(1): 9-15.
      [http://dx.doi.org/10.1590/S1678-77572012000100003] [PMID: 22437671]

[3]   Shiota K. Variability in human embryonic development and its implications for the susceptibility to environmental teratogenesis. Birth Defects Res A Clin Mol Teratol 2009; 85(8): 661-6.
      [http://dx.doi.org/10.1002/bdra.20596] [PMID: 19606457]

[4]   Moore KL, Persaud TV. Embriologia Clínica. Rio de Janeiro: Guanabara Koogan 2000.

[5]   Gorlin RJ, Cohen MM Junior, Levin LS. Teratogenic agents. In: Gorlin RJ, Cohen MM, Hennekam RC, Eds. Syndromes of the head and neck New York. Oxford 1990; pp. 15-31.

[6]   Floyd RL, O'Connor MJ, Sokol RJ, Bertrand J, Cordero JF. Recognition and prevention of fetal alcohol syndrome. Obstet Gynecol 2005; 106(5 Pt 1): 1059-64.
      [http://dx.doi.org/10.1097/01.AOG.0000181822.91205.6f] [PMID: 16260526]

[7]   Zanoti-Jeronymo DV, Nicolau JF, Botti ML, Soares LG. Repercussões do consumo de álcool na gestação – estudo dos efeitos no feto. BJSCR 2014; 6: 40-6.

[8]   Matos SB, Meyer R, Lima FW. Citomegalovírus: Uma revisão da patogenia, epidemiologia e diagnostico da infecção. Rev Saúde Com 2011; 7: 44-57.

[9]   Robertson SE, Featherstone DA, Gacic-Dobo M, Hersh BS. Rubella and congenital rubella syndrome: global update. Rev Panam Salud Publica 2003; 14(5): 306-15.
      [http://dx.doi.org/10.1590/S1020-49892003001000005] [PMID: 14870758]

CHAPTER 4

Dental Management in Rare Facial Clefts

Marcia Ribeiro Gomide*, **Gisele da Silva Dalben*** and **Lucimara Teixeira das Neves***

Bauru School of Dentistry and Hospital for Rehabilitation of Craniofacial Anomalies, University of São Paulo, Brazil

Abstract: The rare facial clefts receive this name due to their low prevalence. The most known and used classification was proposed by Tessier and employs a distinct numbering to indicate clefts affecting the soft and hard tissues, taking as reference point the eyelid and the orbit. The oral characteristics of individuals with rare facial clefts are not specific, and in most cases the oral phenotype follows the structures affected by the defect. Due to the complexity of the cleft and the number of affected structures, the surgical and dental rehabilitation is complex and extensive, requiring the participation of a multi- and interdisciplinary team.

Keywords: Dental care, Orofacial cleft, Phenotype, Tooth abnormalities.

INTRODUCTION

The rare craniofacial clefts present low prevalence and wide spectrum of malformation, affecting both the skull and face in a large variety of manifestations [1]. This diversity of manifestations impairs a universal classification. In an attempt to standardize a terminology for these clefts, Paul Tessier, in 1976, published a clear and simple classification, which has been widely used by the scientific community since then [2].

This classification was initially presented at the International Meeting of Cleft Palate Association, Copenhagen, in August 1973 [1, 2], and is still accepted and used for description of craniofacial and laterofacial clefts because it represents an anatomic system ordered along defined axes, assigning numbers to the several cleft sites, depending on their relationship with the midsagittal plane, in 15

* **Corresponding author Marcia Ribeiro Gomide:** Hospital for Rehabilitation of Craniofacial Anomalies, University of São Paulo, Bauru, Brazil; Tel/Fax: +55 14 3235-8000; E-mail: marcinha@usp.br
* **Gisele da Silva Dalben:** Hospital for Rehabilitation of Craniofacial Anomalies, University of São Paulo, Bauru, Brazil; Tel/Fax: +55 14 3235-8000; E-mail: gsdalben@usp.br
* **Lucimara Teixeira das Neves:** Bauru School of Dentistry and Hospital for Rehabilitation of Craniofacial Anomalies, University of São Paulo, Bauru, Brazil; Tel/Fax: +55 14 3235-8000; E-mail: lucimaraneves@fob.usp.br

locations numbered from 0 to 14, besides including number 30 for the medial mandibular cleft (Fig. **4.1**) [1 - 4].

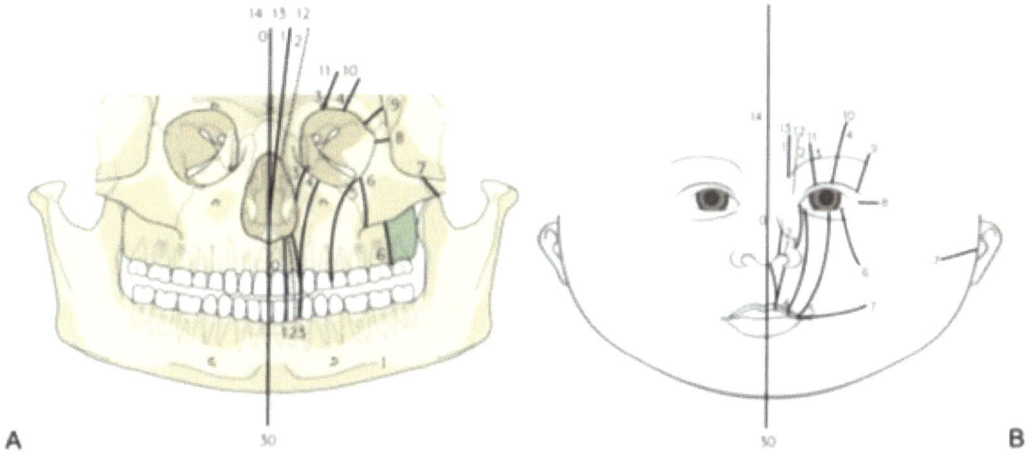

Fig. (4.1). Tessier classification of craniofacial clefts. Source: Ramanathan *et al.,* 2012 [4].

The clefts may affect soft and hard tissues to different extents and in an independent manner. They may occur unilaterally or bilaterally, yet the unilateral clefts are more frequent [1, 2]. The soft tissue anomalies are predominant from the midsagittal plane to the infraorbital foramen, and more severe bone defects are more common from the infraorbital foramen to the temporal bone, except for the ear [3]. It should be highlighted that the vessels and nerves remain unaltered in the soft tissue, even if the bone is absent or hypoplastic due to the clefts [1].

The Tessier classification describes the clefts based on the anatomy of the affected region and considers the eyelids and orbits as reference point, dividing the orbits into two hemispheres for a better understanding. The lower eyelids, together with the cheeks and lip, constitute the southern hemisphere, whose clefts are facial and numbered from 0 to 7. Contralaterally, the upper eyelids constitute the northern hemisphere and clefts at this site are cranial and numbered from 8 to 14. However, the growth centers are not necessarily the same, demanding additional care to define the treatment plan and duration of surgery for cases presenting both cranial and facial clefts. The lines numbering the clefts may have upper (cranial) or lower orientation (facial). The cranial lines have facial correspondents, yet these numbers are different to avoid the erroneous assumption that they necessarily have the same etiopathogenesis [2].

Below, each of these rare craniofacial clefts will be described in detail.

CLEFT #0-14

According to Tessier [2], clefts #0 and 14 represent a median craniofacial dysraphia due to absence of closure of the anterior neuropore. The cleft crosses the frontal bone, giving rise to a "bifid cranium" or a median encephalocele with duplication of the crista galli through the midline, with duplication of the nasal septum, and through the columella, maxilla and lip. The cranial cleft may cause varied degrees of hyperteleorbitism. The occurrence of other milder phenotypic manifestations is possible [5].

CLEFT #1-13

Craniofacial cleft #1 is considered a paramedian cleft; in the soft tissues, the cleft crosses the dome of the alar cartilage (Fig. **4.2**) and occasionally the alveolus and lip, yielding a cleft of the lip and primary palate on the face. It may affect the alar cartilage from a small paramedian notch up to a cleft with structural loss of the nostril. Its cranial correspondent #13 crosses the frontal bone through the olfactory groove of the cribriform plate between the nasal bone and frontal maxillary process, causing hyperteleorbitism and possibly encephalocele [2]. In the soft tissue, the cleft is seen between the eyebrows.

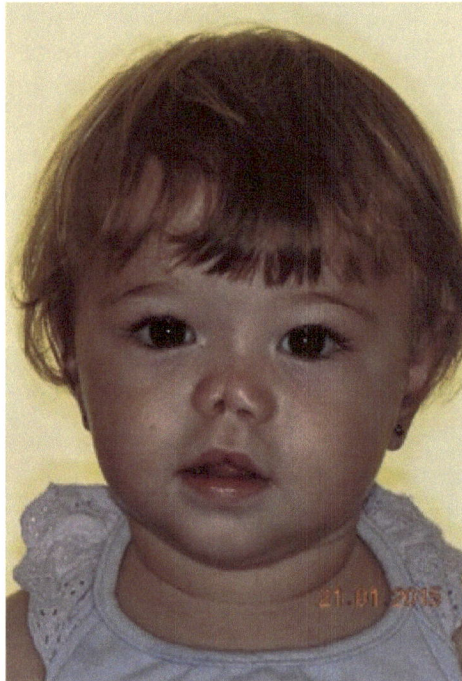

Fig. (4.2). Individual with Tessier cleft #1. To understand the embryogenesis of this cleft, please refer to Figs. (**1.17** and **1.20b**).

CLEFT #2-12

Cleft #2 is paranasal in relation to cleft #1. In the soft tissue, it surrounds the nasal ala between the extremity and the alar cartilage base, manifesting as a typical cleft in the lip. In bone, the cleft crosses the lateral surface of the ethmoid. There may be nose hemiatrophy, supernumerary nostril and lateral proboscis, which are different degrees of the same defect [2]. Cranial cleft #12 displays an increased frontal sinus, exhibiting a coloboma at the eyebrow roots between the nasal bridge and the internal canthi [1].

CLEFT #3-11

Cleft #3 represents the known oculonasal or medial orbito-maxillary cleft, which crosses the lacrimal portion of the lower eyelid. The lacrimal system is obliterated and a coloboma is usually present in the lower eyelid, in addition to more inferior positioning of the medial portion of the canthus. Often there is total absence of the maxillary frontal process and medial wall of the maxillary sinus, which complicates the surgical procedures for rehabilitation.

The cleft extends around the alar base and in the nasolabial groove, with possible presence of a typical cleft lip (Fig. **4.3**). It corresponds to cranial cleft #11, which is an upper medial orbital cleft, with coloboma of the middle third of the upper eyelid, occasionally affecting the eyebrow. There may be some degree of hyperteleorbitism [1, 2].

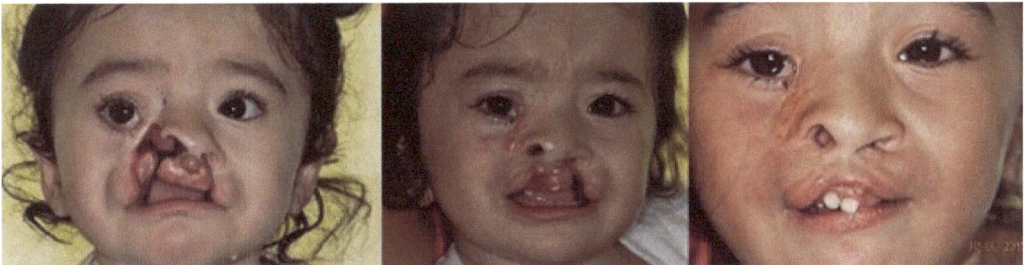

Fig. (4.3). Individual with Tessier cleft #3-11 on the right side and cleft lip and palate on the left side. Notice the evolution after procedures for surgical repair. To understand the embryogenesis of this cleft, please refer to Figs. (**1.17** and **1.22c**).

CLEFT #4-10

Cleft #4, oculofacial cleft I or central orbito-maxillary cleft crosses the lacrimal portion of the lower eyelid almost vertically (Fig. **4.4**), affecting the infraorbital rim and the orbit floor, medially to the infraorbital nerve and through the maxillary sinus, causing sinus extrophy. In severe cases, the clefts may pass through the orbit and there may be anophthalmia (Fig. **4.5**). This cleft is more lateral than #3 and the lacrimal system might be affected. In complete clefts, the skeletal structures present continuity and communication of the mouth with the maxillary sinus and orbit. When bilateral, it distorts the nose and premaxilla in a similar manner as bilateral cleft lip and palate. Its location in the lip and alveolus is the same as typical cleft lip and palate.

Cleft #10 affects the middle third of the supraorbital rim laterally to the supraorbital nerve (Fig. **4.6**). It extends to the orbit floor and frontal bone, possibly causing encephalocele. There may be coloboma of the middle third of the upper eyelid and the eyebrow may be divided into two portions [1, 2].

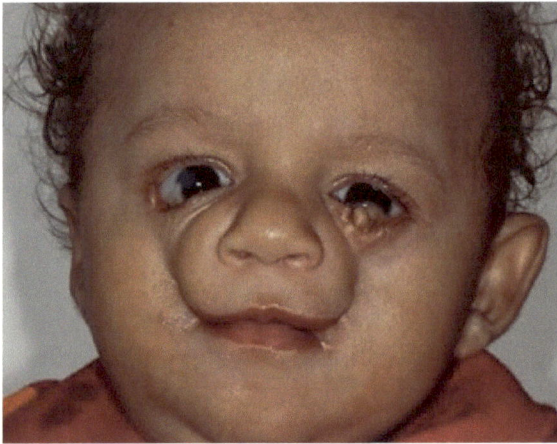

Fig. (4.4). Individual with bilateral Tessier cleft #4. To understand the embryogenesis of this cleft, please refer to Fig. (**1.17**).

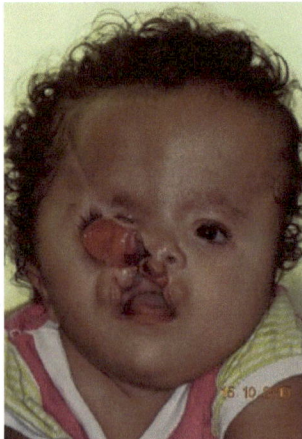

Fig. (4.5). Individual with Tessier cleft #4 on the right side and cleft lip on the left side. Notice the anophthalmia and the cleft line extending through the frontal bone, dividing the eyelid and eyebrow into two sections. To understand the embryogenesis of this cleft, please refer to Fig. (**1.17**), observing the line describing cleft #4.

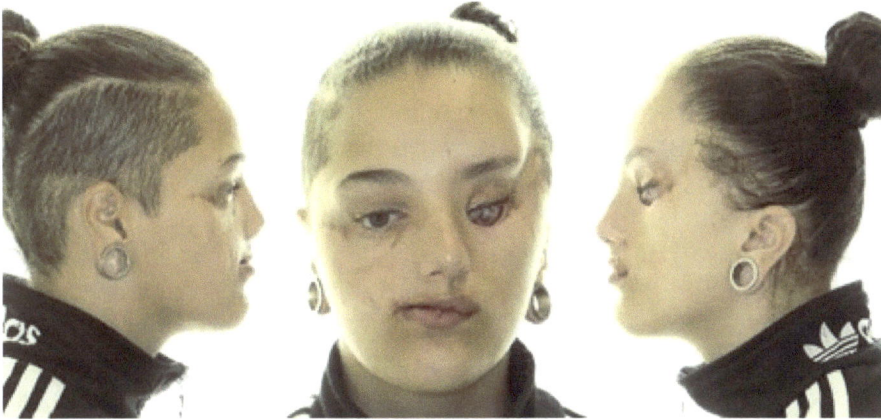

Fig. (4.6). Individual with Tessier cleft #4. To understand the embryogenesis of this cleft, please refer to Fig. (**1.17**).

CLEFT #5-9

Cleft #5 was known as oculofacial cleft II or lateral orbito-maxillary cleft. It extends from the region close to the commissure up to the middle third of the lower eyelid, or between the medial and lateral thirds, affecting the cheek as a groove (Fig. **4.7**). It crosses the infraorbital rim, orbit floor and maxilla laterally to the infraorbital nerve and maxillary sinus, extending through the alveolus posterior to the canine, at the premolar region. This is the rarest among all oblique facial clefts. Cleft #9 is an upper lateral orbital cleft that affects the lateral third of the upper eyelid and the supralateral orbital angle. Very few cases have been described in the literature [1, 2].

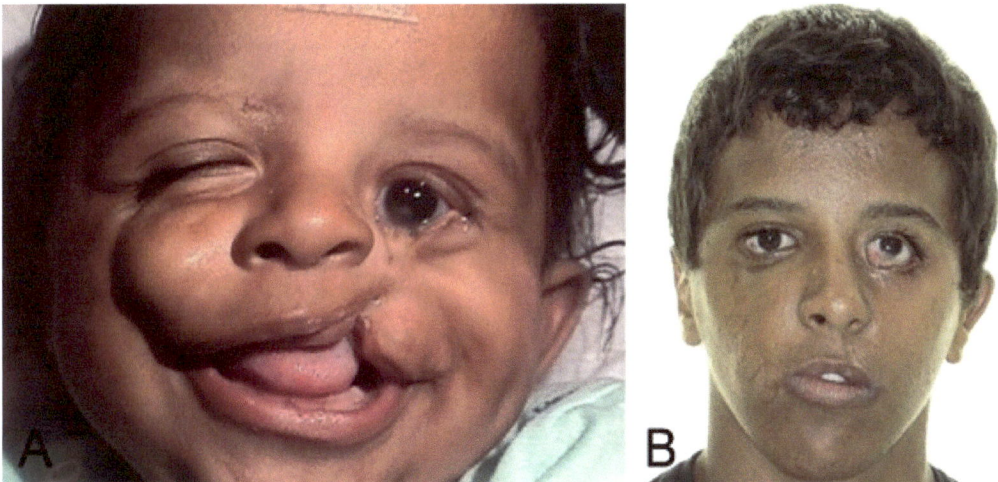

Fig. (4.7). Individual with Tessier cleft #5 on the right side and #4 on the left side, as a baby (A) and in adolescence (B). To understand the embryogenesis of this cleft, please refer to Figs (**1.17** and **1.24**).

CLEFT #6

Cleft #6 is a maxillary-zygomatic cleft with coloboma of the lower eyelid between the middle and lateral thirds; it separates the maxilla from the zygomatic bone, opening the infraorbital cleft. The posterior aspect of the maxilla is short, with high-arched palate and choanal atresia. It may affect the alveolus and present a vertical groove on the cheek, which may be more or less marked, similar to a scar. It may occur in combination with cleft #5. This cleft has been widely accepted as a variation of expressivity in the phenotypic spectrum of Treacher Collins syndrome. In these cases, the deformity includes coloboma in the middle third of the lower eyelid and downslanting palpebral fissures. The ears may be prominent or normal in most cases, yet some hearing impairment may be present. Bone defects occur at the region of zygomaticomaxillary suture and are characterized by the presence of a typical cleft or hypoplasia of the bone tissue, yet maintaining the zygomatic arch intact. Occasionally, hair may be observed at the malar region.

CLEFT #7

Cleft #7 is a temporozygomatic cleft that usually causes absence of the zygomatic arch and deformities in the mandibular ramus, condyle and coronoid process. The maxilla is short in the vertical plane and the alveolus may be hypoplastic. The soft tissue anomalies include ear malformations and hypoplasia or absence of the temporal muscle. It is the most lateral facial cleft, being considered facial and cranial. Its facial manifestations include macrostomia (with the cleft extending up to the commissure) (Figs. **4.8**, **4.9** and **4.10**) and preauricular tags. It may be unilateral or bilateral, with predominance of unilateral cases. It is one of the most common and known rare facial clefts [6]. It is also described as hemifacial microsomia, microtia, otomandibular dysostosis, 1st and 2nd pharyngeal arch cleft, and others. For further information, please refer to Chapter 7.

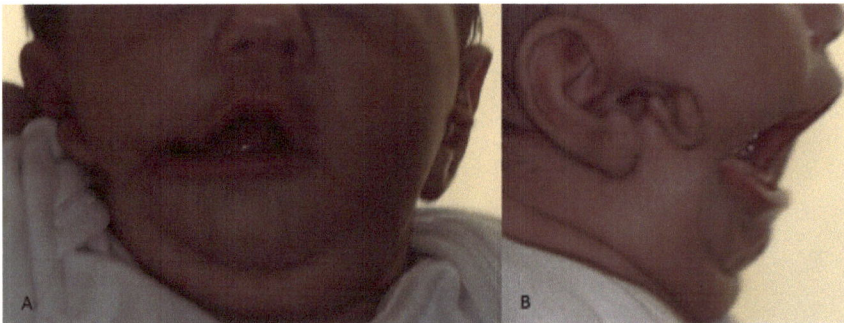

Fig. (4.8). Individual with Tessier cleft #7 on the right side with preauricular tags. To understand the embryogenesis of this cleft, please refer to Figs. (**1.17** and **1.24**).

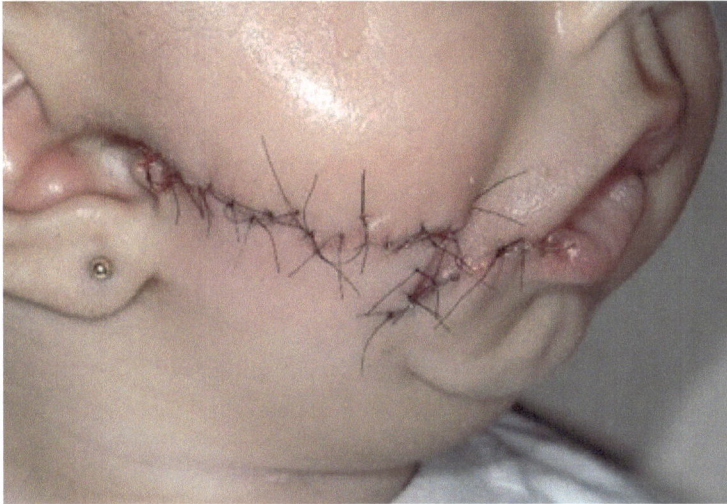

Fig. (4.9). Postoperative view of the same individual presented in Fig. **4.11**. To understand the embryogenesis of this cleft, please refer to Figs. (**1.17** and **1.24**).

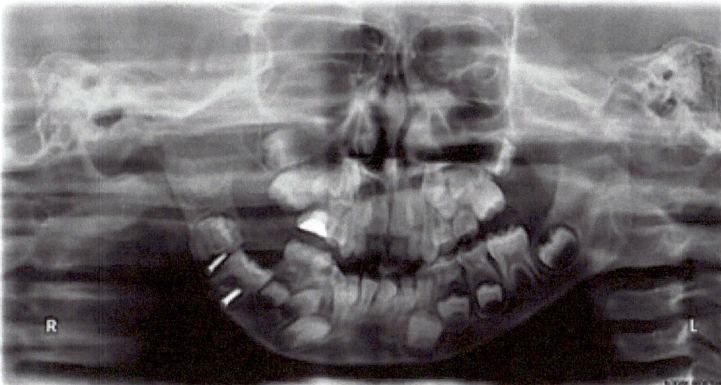

Fig. (4.10). Panoramic radiograph of the same individual presented in Figs. (**4.8, 4.9**). This individual presented severe micrognathia with airway disorders and required distraction osteogenesis at an early age. The radiograph evidences the marked mandibular asymmetry, with smaller dimensions on the side affected by the cleft; also notice the screws used for distraction osteogenesis, which affected the permanent mandibular right first molar. This complication may occur and cannot be prevented due to the early age when distraction osteogenesis is performed. For further information on distraction osteogenesis, please refer to Chapter 9.

CLEFT #8

Cleft #8 is a frontozygomatic cleft, corresponding to facial cleft #6. In several cases, a piece of zygomatic bone has been found attached to the sphenoid tubercle, without relationship with the maxilla or frontal or temporal bones, in which three prominences were identified, interpreted as representing the three growth centers of the maxillary bone that had not merged with the three surrounding bones. In the absence of zygomatic bone, sesamoid bones have been found in the aponeurosis common to the temporal and masseter bones. This rare cleft corresponds to a loss of continuity with the canthi, extending to the temporal region. When the underlying bones are affected, it presents as a cleft in the frontozygomatic suture.

Clefts #6, 7 and 8 may appear together in individuals with Treacher Collins/Franceschetti syndrome. In these cases the zygomatic bone is absent, there is coloboma of the lower eyelid and the ears present inferior positioning or reduced size.

CLEFT #30

This is an isolated and very rare cleft, with 4 to 5 cases at every 1,000,000. It does not present hereditary characteristics nor gender predilection. In cases of severe clefts, the hyoid and sternum bone may be affected [7]. It involves the lower lip and may affect the mandibular alveolar bone or not, as well as the tongue. This is affected in nearly 35% of cases. Ankyloglossia is present in almost all cases. There are also reports of cardiac and limb malformations, among others, associated with cleft #30 [7].

ORAL FEATURES IN INDIVIDUALS WITH RARE FACIAL CLEFTS

Individuals with rare facial clefts usually do not present specific dental manifestations; rather, they may present orodental alterations directly related with the anatomical disorders caused by the facial clefts. It should be considered that the physical appearance may lead to a mistaken judgment of intellectual disability in these individuals. Thus, the dental professional should achieve information about the neuropsychomotor development of each individual and assess the conditions for compliance. According to the literature, the major dental involvement in individuals with rare facial clefts is related with the presence of occlusal disorders caused by the defect, especially when the bone tissue is affected [4]. When necessary, the dental and orthodontic treatment may be performed as usual. In some cases, active orthodontic treatment may be necessary preoperatively for bone repositioning; however, this is not a routine procedure [8, 9].

As previously mentioned, adequate treatment requires knowledge on individuals and their ability for compliance, as well as on the oral manifestations caused by the anatomical disorder. The phenotype of individuals with cleft #0 is widely variable both extra- and intraorally, yet some cases with this cleft may present significant interincisal diastema or anterior open bite, from both esthetic and functional standpoints. In cases with clefts #1, 2, 3 and 4, the oral disorders are usually related with clefts affecting the alveolar ridge, *i.e.* teeth close to the anatomical defect, especially the maxillary lateral incisors, may present abnormalities of shape, structure and position. In individuals with clefts #5 associated with #6 and #7, there have been reports of multiple supernumerary teeth in the posterior maxillary region [4, 6]. In the presence of cleft #7, which is more common, there is also a report of dentigerous cyst in the maxilla at the side affected by the cleft [10]. Cases of macrostomia with bone involvement require clinical and radiographic evaluation for dental and orthodontic intervention as needed.

The rehabilitation of individuals with rare facial clefts may require orthognathic surgery in addition to dental and orthodontic intervention; for that purpose, the maxillofacial surgeon should perform adequate clinical and radiographic diagnosis, including additional diagnostic means if necessary. It should be highlighted that the rehabilitation of individuals with rare facial clefts should be individualized and, above all, respect the individual's expectations [11].

CONFLICT OF INTEREST

The author (editor) declares no conflict of interest, financial or otherwise.

ACKNOWLEDGEMENTS

Declared none.

REFERENCES

[1]   Cirurjanos Plástikos Mundi. Rare Cranio-Facial clefts Available at: http://www.cpmundi.org/ adjuntos/manuales/es/rare_cranio-facial_clefts-5.pdf

[2]   Tessier P. Anatomical classification facial, cranio-facial and latero-facial clefts. J Maxillofac Surg 1976; 4(2): 69-92.
        [http://dx.doi.org/10.1016/S0301-0503(76)80013-6] [PMID: 820824]

[3]   Gorlin RJ, Cohen MM Jr, Levin LS. Syndromes of the head and neck. New York: Oxford University 1990.

[4]   Ramanathan M, Parameswaran A, Jayakumar N, Sneha P, Sailer HF. A rare case of multiple oblique facial clefts with supernumerary teeth: case report. Craniomaxillofac Trauma Reconstr 2012; 5(4): 239-42.
        [http://dx.doi.org/10.1055/s-0032-1329541] [PMID: 24294408]

[5]   Guruprasad Y, Chauhan DS. Midline nasal dermoid cyst with Tessier's 0 cleft. J Nat Sci Biol Med 2014; 5(2): 479-82.
        [http://dx.doi.org/10.4103/0976-9668.136272] [PMID: 25097442]

[6]   Hou M, Liu C, Wang J, Zhang L, Gao Q. Lateral or oblique facial clefts associated with accessory maxillae: Review of the literature and report of a case. J Craniomaxillofac Surg 2015; 43(5): 585-92.
        [http://dx.doi.org/10.1016/j.jcms.2015.02.008] [PMID: 25862344]

[7]   Tafreshi M, Aminolsharieh Najafi S, Hasheminejad R, Mirfazeli A, Shafiee A. Tessier number 30 clefts with congenital heart defects. Iran Red Crescent Med J 2015; 17(3): e19078.
        [http://dx.doi.org/10.5812/ircmj.19078] [PMID: 26019899]

[8]   Maeda T, Oyama A, Okamoto T, *et al.* Combination of Tessier clefts 3 and 4: case report of a rare anomaly with 12 years' follow-up. J Craniomaxillofac Surg 2014; 42(8): 1985-9.
         [http://dx.doi.org/10.1016/j.jcms.2014.09.003] [PMID: 25441869]

[9]   Spolyar JL, Hnatiuk M, Shaheen KW, *et al.* Tessier No. 3 and No. 4 clefts: Sequential treatment in infancy by pre-surgical orthopedic skeletal contraction, comprehensive reconstruction, and novel surgical lengthening of the ala base-canthal distance. J Craniomaxillofac Surg 2015; 43(7): 1261-8.
         [http://dx.doi.org/10.1016/j.jcms.2015.06.002] [PMID: 26170000]

[10]   Issar Y, Kaushal N, Goomer P. Unusual case of concomitant occurrence of Tessier's number 7 cleft and dentigerous cyst. Contemp Clin Dent 2014; 5(3): 402-5.
         [http://dx.doi.org/10.4103/0976-237X.137972] [PMID: 25191083]

[11]   Allam KA, Lim AA, Elsherbiny A, Kawamoto HK. The Tessier number 3 cleft: a report of 10 cases and review of literature. J Plast Reconstr Aesthet Surg 2014; 67(8): 1055-62.
         [http://dx.doi.org/10.1016/j.bjps.2014.04.020] [PMID: 24933239]

CHAPTER 5

Syndromes with Orofacial Clefts

Beatriz Costa[*], Cleide Felício de Carvalho Carrara[*] and Vivian de Agostino Biella Passos[*]

Hospital for Rehabilitation of Craniofacial Anomalies, University of São Paulo; University of Sagrado Coração, Brazil

Abstract: Orofacial clefts are among the commonest malformations affecting mankind; even though most cases of orofacial clefts are non-syndromic, they may also manifest concomitantly with a wide array of syndromes. These syndromes with orofacial clefts often also cause diverse tooth abnormalities; knowledge on these peculiarities is fundamental for professionals to allow proper dental care for affected individuals.

Keywords: Dental care, Ectrodactyly, Ectodermal dysplasia, and cleft-lip-palate syndrome, Holoprosencephaly, Orofacial cleft, Orofaciodigital syndromes, Rapp-Hodgkin syndrome, Pierre Robin syndrome, Richieri Costa Pereira syndrome, Tooth abnormalities, Van der Woude syndrome, 22q11 deletion syndrome.

HOLOPROSENCEPHALY

Holoprosencephaly (HPE) is a structural brain anomaly occurring during the third and fourth weeks of pregnancy, caused by incomplete cleavage of the forebrain into right and left hemispheres [1, 2], thus the name *holoprosencephaly* (Greek: *holos* – whole; *prosencephalon* – forebrain). It is the most common defect of the forebrain and middle face in humans [3], affecting 1 in every 16,000 livebirths and approximately 1 in every 200 spontaneous miscarriages [4]. It may be associated with genetic syndromes, especially the Smith-Lemli-Opitz syndrome. In relatively rare cases, subgroups of individuals may present additional structural brain malformations, such as schizencephaly of extracerebral manifestations as ectrodactyly (refer to the EEC syndrome later in this chapter for a clinical image of this malformation), radial limb defects, agnathia or craniosynostosis [4].

[*] **Corresponding author Beatriz Costa:** Hospital for Rehabilitation of Craniofacial Anomalies, University of São Paulo, Bauru, Brazil; Tel/Fax: +55 14 3235-8000; E-mail: biacosta@usp.br
[*] **Cleide Felício de Carvalho Carrara:** Hospital for Rehabilitation of Craniofacial Anomalies, University of São Paulo, Bauru, Brazil; Tel/Fax: +55 14 3235-8000; E-mail: cleidecarrara@usp.br
[*] **Vivian de Agostino Biella Passos:** University of Sagrado Coração, Bauru, Brazil; Tel/Fax: +55 14 2107-7000; E-mail: vivibiella@hotmail.com

Gisele da Silva Dalben & Marcia Ribeiro Gomide (Eds.)

HPE may be associated with a myriad of craniofacial anomalies, including cyclopia, microcephaly, hypoteleorbitism, depressed nasal bridge, single maxillary incisor, and cleft lip with or without cleft palate (CLP). Some affected individuals also present pituitary dysfunction and feeding disorders [1].

The etiology of both syndromic and non-syndromic HPE is heterogeneous. It is related with genes 21q22.3 and 2q37.1-q37.3 [2]. Chromosomal abnormalities are present in up to 50% of individuals with HPE and may include trisomy 13, trisomy 18, and several other variations in the number of copies [1]. The disorder presents autosomal recessive inheritance, yet autosomal dominant inheritance has been observed in some cases, whose widely variable phenotype is related with a locus on distal 7q.

Among the environmental aspects, gestational diabetes is highlighted, with a prevalence of 1-2% among children of diabetic mothers, which is considered a significant finding [5]. The utilization of folic acid in pregnancy seems to have a protective effect [6]. There are contradictory and inconsistent reports concerning possible associations between HPE and respiratory diseases, anemia, smoking and utilization of salicylates, antiepileptic drugs, sexual hormones, statins and alcohol [7].

The phenotype of HPE is variable between simple cases and between members of a same family with hereditary manifestation of HPE; consequently, subtle facial characteristics may be neglected in members of affected families. If any child is diagnosed with HPE, the first-degree relatives should be questioned and examined to identify individuals with microcephaly, hypoteleorbitism, or single maxillary incisor.

Since some cases of HPE present autosomal dominant inheritance, the identification of other family members that may be affected influences the indication of genetic tests and identification of risk factors [1].

The typical facies of holoprosencephaly (Fig. **5.1**) is observed in approximately 80% of cases. It is characterized by cyclopia or more commonly by hypoteleorbitism, associated with agenesis of nasal bones, median cleft lip with or without cleft palate (Fig. **5.2**) and severe neurological disorders, with short life expectancy. Thus, the treatment of holoprosencephaly should comprise a careful risk-benefit analysis [8].

Some authors have reported correlation between holoprosencephaly and the presence of a single median maxillary central incisor (Figs. **5.3** and **5.4**) [9 - 11], which may affect both the deciduous and permanent dentitions [2], whose inheritance is related with chromosomal region 7q36 [12]. Thus, the presence of a single median maxillary central incisor in an adult may constitute a risk factor to holoprosencephaly in the offspring, warranting genetic counseling for family planning.

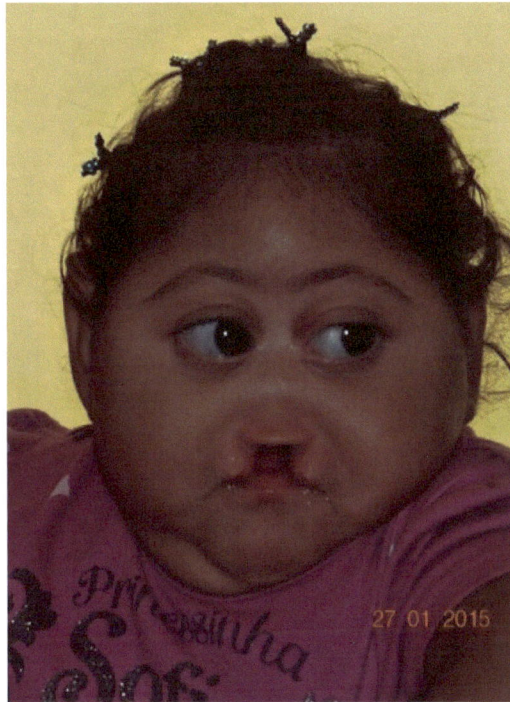

Fig. (5.1). Individual with holoprosencephaly. Notice the hypoteleorbitism and depressed nasal bridge.

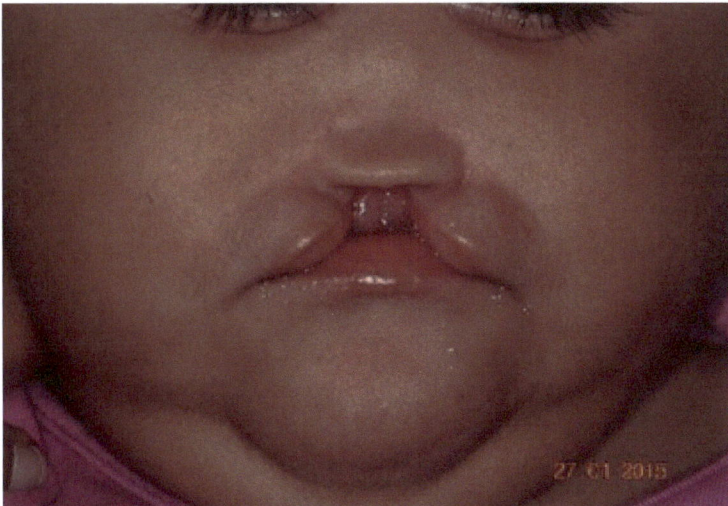

Fig. (5.2). Closer view of individual in Fig. (**5.1**), evidencing the median cleft lip.

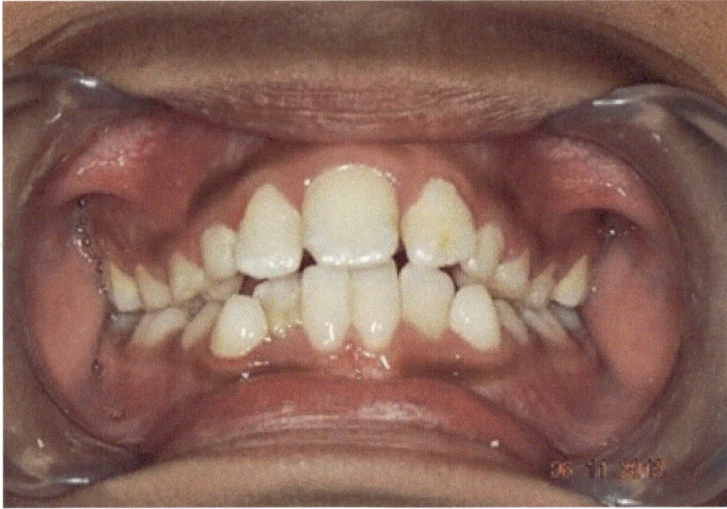

Fig. (5.3). Individual with single median maxillary central incisor. Notice that the central incisor is located exactly in the midline and presents increased mesiodistal diameter. This disorder must be carefully differentiated from agenesis of a central incisor, in which the present central incisor would not be positioned in the midline and would present normal mesiodistal diameter.

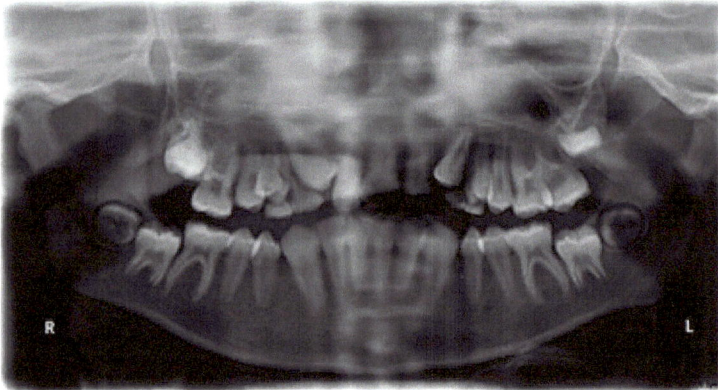

Fig. (5.4). Panoramic radiograph of the case presented in Fig. **(5.3)**.

VAN DER WOUDE SYNDROME

The Van der Woude syndrome (VWS) was initially described by Demarquay in 1845 [13, 14]. Even though VWS was reported by Demarquay, the syndrome was named after Anne Van der Woude, who extensively described the syndrome in 1954 [15]. Van der Woude was the first to report the combination of congenital lower lip pits with cleft lip and/or cleft palate, introducing a new clinical disorder and also describing its mode of inheritance.

The prevalence of the syndrome ranges from 1.65/100,000 [16] to 1/ 75,000 – 1/100,000 inhabitants [17]. According to Rizos and Spyropoulos [15], the VWS affects both genders, with predilection for the female gender.

The VWS is the most common syndrome among individuals with cleft lip and palate and accounts for 2% of all cases [18]. The phenotypic expression of clefts ranges from cleft lip with or without cleft palate, incomplete unilateral cleft lip, isolated cleft palate, submucous cleft palate, bifid uvula, up to complete bilateral cleft lip and palate [15] (Figs. **5.5** and **5.6**).

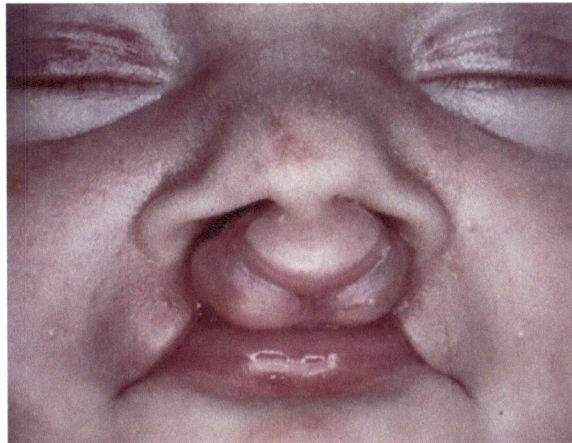

Fig. (5.5). Congenital lower lip pits and complete bilateral cleft lip and palate in child with Van der Woude syndrome.

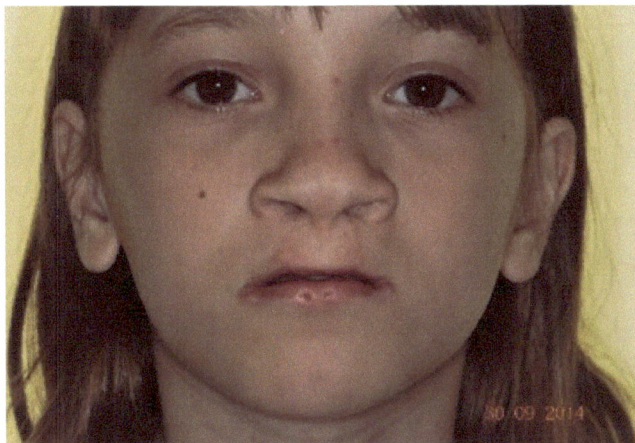

Fig. (5.6). Congenital lower lip pits and repaired complete bilateral cleft lip and palate in the same child, at an older age. Surgery is often necessary in the lower lip to enhance the esthetics.

Pits or conical elevations in the lower lip (microform) are present in 80% [19] to 88% of cases [15]. The pits are usually bilateral, yet they may also occur unilaterally or at the center of the lower lip vermillion. The depth of depressions is variable, reaching up to 25 millimeters, with round or slightly flattened openings, which may communicate with the mixed acinar gland ducts. Other clinical variant is the microform, which presents only as conical paramedian elevations or prominences [20].

A study revealed that lower lip pits are associated with clefts in nearly half of individuals, among which two thirds presented cleft lip or cleft lip and palate and one third had isolated cleft palate, which is similar to the proportion observed for individuals with non-syndromic clefts [19]. In other study, approximately 33% of individuals with lower lip pits did not have clefts, 33% presented lower lip pits with cleft lip and palate, and 33% of individuals exhibited pits with cleft palate or submucous cleft palate [21].

The wide variability of phenotypic expression in VWS was described by Jobling [22], who presented a confirmed case of monozygotic twins (MZ), both affected by VWS due to a mutation in the IRF6 gene, yet with markedly different phenotype. This report provided evidence that MZ twins with VWS may have discordant phenotypes, probably due to modifying factors. Lower lip pits were present in both twins, yet only one exhibited cleft lip and palate. This demonstrates the complexity of phenotype expression of VWS and highlights the need of further studies on modifying genes, genetic factors that are related with the intrauterine environment and environmental factors that may also play a role in the etiology of hypodontia.

Concerning the etiology, the VWS is an autosomal dominant disorder with high penetrance and widely variable expressivity, characterized by the presence of congenital lower lip pits, associated or not with cleft lip and/or palate and hypodontia. By molecular genetic studies, investigators have identified the gene IRF6 in chromosome 1, located at the critical region 1q32-p41, as being responsible for VWS [23].

Most cases present variable intrafamilial expression, and nearly complete penetrance is observed in 80 to 97% of cases [24]. However, penetrance of 97% to 100% was reported when hypodontia and submucous cleft palate were included as manifestations of the syndrome [20].

Concerning the dental aspects, hypodontia in VWS is observed in 10-20% [19] to 75% of cases [25]. According to Cervenka and Gorlin [24] and Calzavara Pinton *et al.,* [26], a close relationship was observed between the syndrome and congenital absence of second premolars; however, Rizos and Spyropoulos [16] also associated the second molar and lateral incisor.

VELOCARDIOFACIAL SYNDROME

The velocardiofacial syndrome affects nearly 1 in every 2,000 to 5,000 livebirths [27]. It is among the commonest syndromes with multiple anomalies, yet it is still underdiagnosed [27].

This syndrome presents autosomal dominant inheritance related with the chromosomal region 22q11, with variable expressivity and predominance of maternal inheritance [28].

The syndrome is characterized by cleft palate, learning disorders, typical facies (Fig. **5.7**) with prominent nose and mandibular retrusion, and cardiovascular anomalies. It may also comprise breathing disorders, short stature, microcephaly, intellectual impairment, mild ear anomalies and inguinal hernia. It may be associated with Robin sequence and velopharyngeal insufficiency [29, 30]. According to the study of Ryan *et al.,* [28] on 558 individuals with velocardiofacial syndrome, 9% of cases presented cleft palate, 32% velopharyngeal insufficiency, 60% hypocalcemia, 75% heart problems and 36% kidney abnormalities.

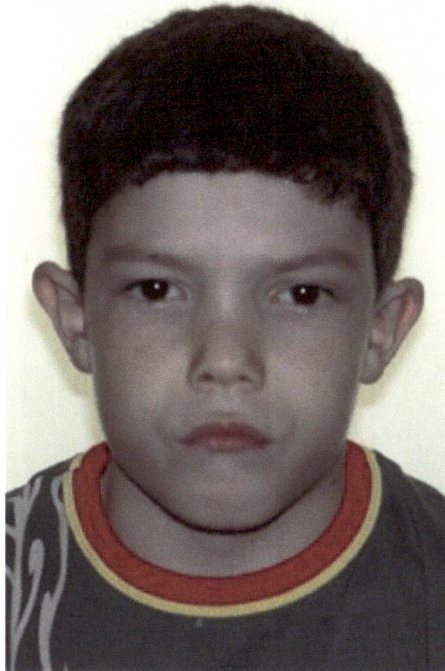

Fig. (5.7). Typical facies in individual with velocardiofacial syndrome.

Dental anomalies are observed in most individuals. The study of Dalben *et al.,* [29] revealed that 76.92% presented at least one tooth abnormality, with predominance of hypoplastic disorders, mainly hypodevelopment of the lingual cusp of the mandibular first premolar (Fig. **5.8**) and enamel opacities (Fig. **5.9**).

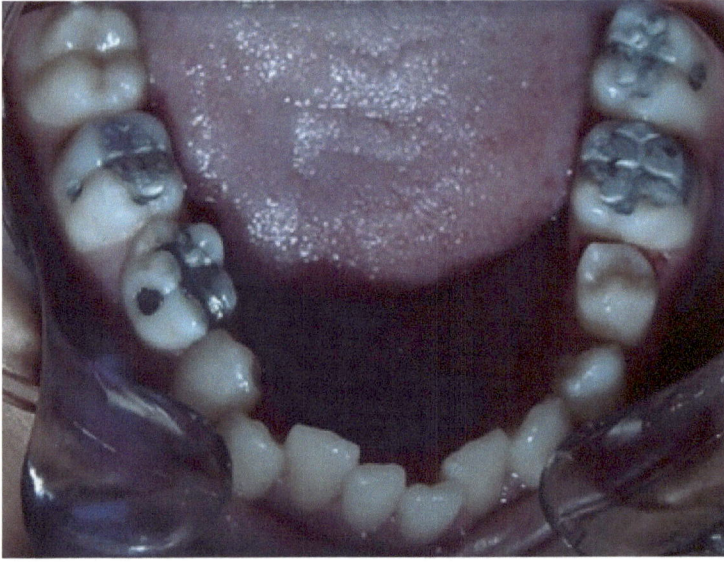

Fig. (5.8). Hypodevelopment of the lingual cusp of both mandibular first premolars in individual with velocardiofacial syndrome.

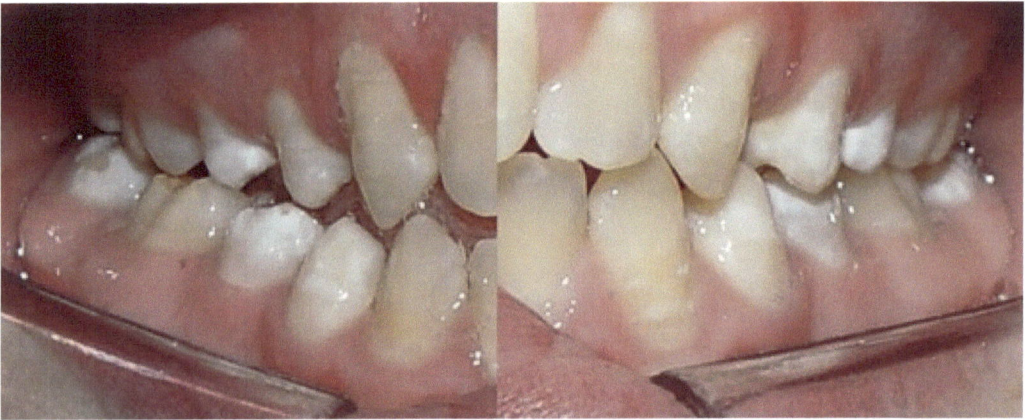

Fig. (5.9). Generalized enamel opacities in individual with velocardiofacial syndrome.

From a clinical standpoint, oral health maintenance is fundamental because the high prevalence of enamel disorders associated with low salivary flow may increase the occurrence of caries in these individuals [31]. In turn, professionals should be attentive to possible systemic involvement, performing careful anamnesis, and to the neurological development of each individual, to check the possibility of compliance before any dental intervention [32], as well as the possible cardiovascular involvement for prevention of bacterial endocarditis.

OROFACIODIGITAL SYNDROME

The orofaciodigital syndrome is a rare condition with high phenotypic variability, possibly presenting 13 subtypes [33]. Type I is the most common (OFD I), which is characterized by congenital malformations of the oral cavity, face, digits, and central nervous system. The estimated prevalence is 1/50,000 to 1/150,000 livebirths [34], and is characterized as an X-linked dominant (chromosomal region Xp22.3-p22.2), thereby it affects only females and is lethal to males, leading to spontaneous abortion, except for individuals with Klinefelter syndrome (XXY).

Malformations of the central nervous system characteristic of OFD 1 include agenesis of the corpus callosum, intracerebral epithelial or arachnoidal cysts, porencephaly, grey matter heterotopia, cerebellum malformations, and abnormal gyral formations [35].

The overall clinical characteristics commonly include hand malformations (syndactyly, clinodactyly, brachydactyly and occasionally postaxial polydactyly) (Fig. **5.10**), renal cyst, intellectual disability, short stature, hearing impairment, telecanthus and hyperteleorbitism, alopecia and facial asymmetry [36, 37].

The typical facies of orofaciodigital syndrome is represented by hypertele-orbitism, miliaria, alopecia, facial asymmetry, alar hypoplasia, micrognathia and low-set ears [38, 39] (Figs. **5.10** and **5.11**).

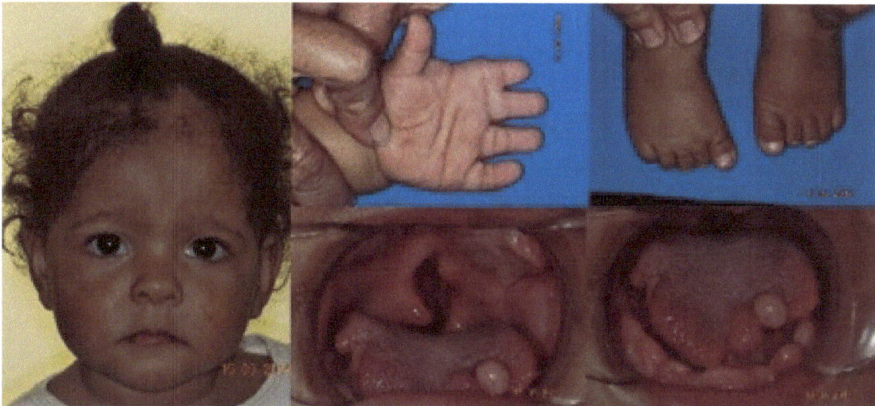

Fig. (5.10). Miliaria on the face, brachydactyly of the hands and feet, cleft palate and multiple tongue hamartomas in individual with orofaciodigital syndrome.

The oral characteristics comprise hyperplastic lingual frenum with ankyloglossia, atrophy of the upper lip frenum [37], tongue hamartomas observed in 70% of cases [40] (Fig. **5.11**), bifid or lobulated tongue (Fig. **5.11**), small median cleft of the upper lip, cleft palate, and high-arched palate. Dental anomalies comprise supernumerary teeth or hypodontia, double teeth, enamel hypoplasia and caries susceptibility [36, 41 - 43].

The study of Tagliani *et al.,* [37] revealed 100% of individuals with OFD I in their sample exhibited dental anomalies, including agenesis of the mandibular permanent lateral incisor (75%), either isolated or combined with agenesis of other teeth; supernumerary teeth (100%), enamel hypoplasia of permanent incisors (58.3%), tooth rotation (41.6%), anterior open bite, high-arched palate and multiple buccal frena (100%) (Fig. **5.11**).

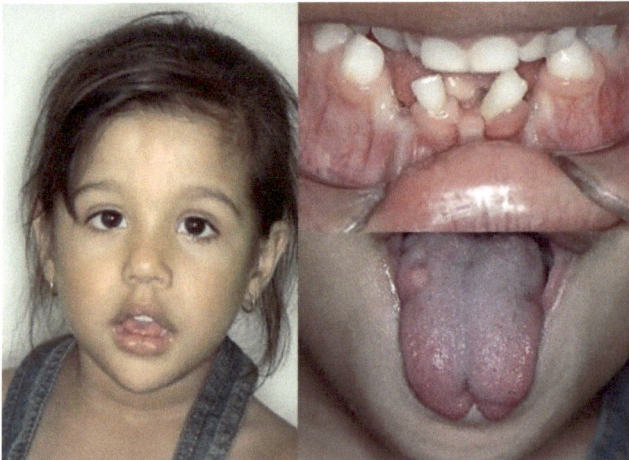

Fig. (5.11). Facial aspect, multiple buccal frena promoting "notches" in the mandibular arch, hypodontia of deciduous mandibular lateral incisors, bifid tongue and tongue hamartoma in individual with orofaciodigital syndrome.

The esthetic and functional involvement inherent to the syndrome and its influence in each individual should be observed. Due to the variable intellectual disability, the dental treatment should consider the cognitive capacity of each individual, besides emphasis on the prevention of oral diseases, due to the possibly difficult compliance.

EEC SYNDROME

The EEC syndrome is a rare autosomal dominant disorder, yet some cases of autosomal recessive inheritance have been reported [44]. It may be associated with more than 170 different syndromes [45].

Most cases of EEC syndrome (90%) are caused by mutations in the TP63 gene [17, 45 - 49]. EEC is one of the five different ectodermal dysplasia syndromes caused by mutations in this gene, namely acro-dermato-ungual-lacrimal-tooth syndrome (ADULT, OMIM 103285), ankyloblepharon-ectodermal defects-cleft lip/palate syndrome (AEC, OMIM 106260), limb-mammary syndrome (LMS, OMIM 603543), and Rapp-Hodgkin syndrome (RHS, OMIM 129400) [46]. The most common syndromes within this group are hypohidrotic and hidrotic ectodermal dysplasias [45].

More than 300 cases have been described in the literature, affecting both male and female genders [45], with a prevalence of 1 in 90,000 in the general population [48]. In rare cases, individuals with EEC syndrome present chromosomal alterations in the long arm of chromosome 7q11.2-q21.3 [44, 45]. In individuals with clinical characteristics suggesting the diagnosis of EEC syndrome, the initial physical examination should prioritize analysis of mutation in the TP63 gene [48].

Clinical diagnosis may be complicated by the widely variable expressivity [47, 48, 50 - 52]. The EEC syndrome is characterized by limb malformations with ectrodactyly ("lobster claw"), ectodermal dysplasia and cleft lip and palate (Figs. **5.12**, **5.13** and **5.14**). Tissues of ectodermal origin are affected, the defects are characterized as developmental anomalies, and heredity is strongly related [45]. Ectrodactyly affects both hands and feet in 90% of cases (Figs. **5.13** and **5.14**) and may be diagnosed prenatally by ultrasound, yet the presence of one normal hand and syndactyly (fusion between two or more fingers or toes, involving soft and/or hard tissues, called cutaneous syndactyly and synostosis, respectively) has been reported in some cases [46, 53].

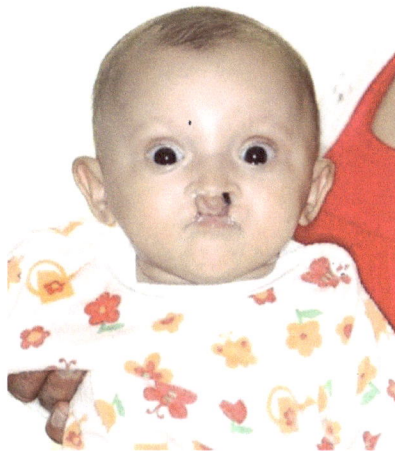

Fig. (5.12). Facial aspect of child with EEC syndrome.

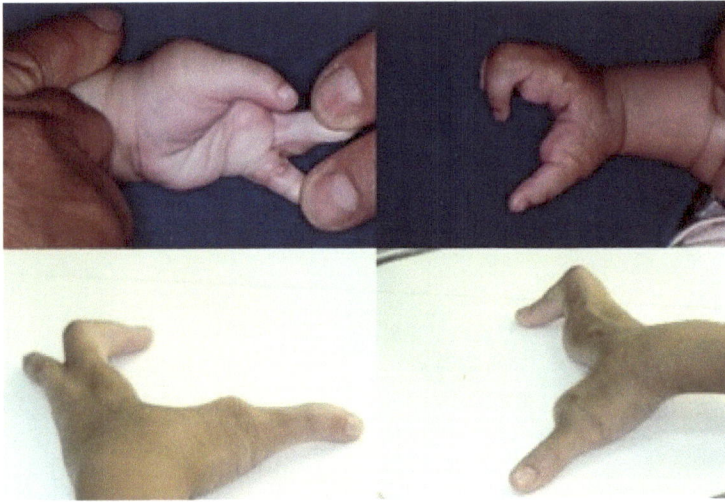

Fig. (5.13). Ectrodactyly of both hands in the individual presented in Fig. (**5.12**), as a baby and at an older age.

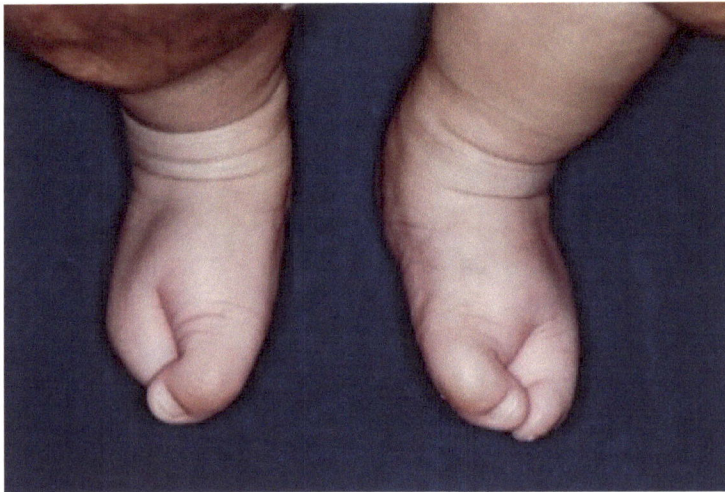

Fig. (5.14). Ectrodactyly of both feet in the same individual presented in Figs. (**5.12** and **5.13**).

Ectodermal dysplasia may manifest with keratoconjunctivitis, nasolacrimal duct abnormalities, dry or eczematous skin, sparse hair, nail dystrophy, tooth abnormalities as hypodontia, anodontia and alterations in the shape and mineralized structure of teeth [48] (Figs. **5.15** and **5.16**). The hair and skin usually present hypopigmentation, except in Black individuals. Microcephaly and intellectual disability may be present in few cases [21, 44].

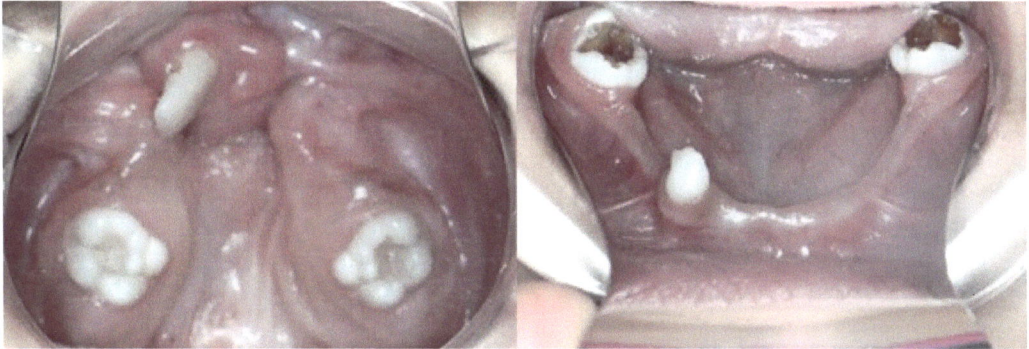

Fig. (5.15). Tooth abnormalities of number and structure in the same individual presented in Figs. (**5.12** to **5.14**) – clinical aspect.

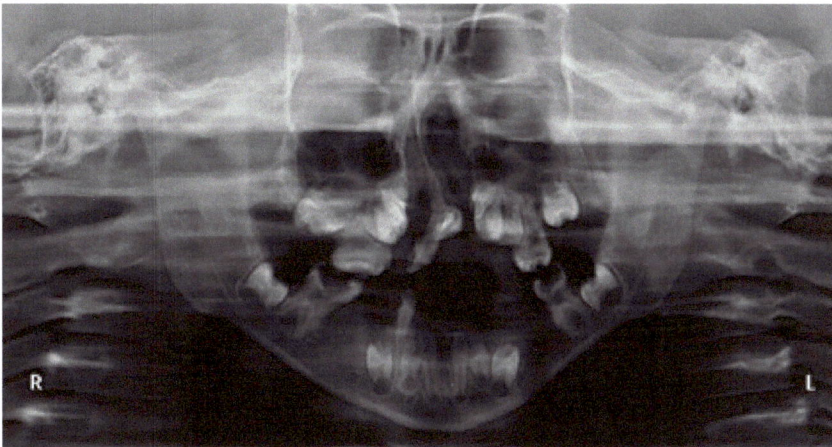

Fig. (5.16). Tooth abnormalities of number and structure in the same individual presented in Figs. (**5.12** to **5.14**) – radiographic aspect.

Individuals with EEC may present cleft lip with or without cleft palate, as well as isolated cleft palate. Both present hereditary pattern with variable expressivity. Cleft lip and palate, usually bilateral, is observed in nearly 75% of cases, with possibility of isolated cleft palate in 210% and absence of cleft in others. Tooth abnormalities as hypodontia of deciduous and permanent teeth, hypodontia, microdontia, peg-shaped teeth, enamel alterations as hypoplasias and opacities are common. The reduced maxillary dimensions favor the occurrence of anterior and posterior crossbite [21, 45, 48, 54 - 57].

Xerostomia may be present, due to the possible atresia or absence of the parotid duct [21, 44]. The literature cites radiographic evidence of widening of the coronal pulp chamber and root canals in molars (taurodontism) [50]. The combination of these factors, as well as the presence of limb deformities that impair the adequate oral hygiene, increases the caries susceptibility in individuals with EEC syndrome. Case reports evidence high caries prevalence affecting most or all present teeth, thus the need of regular prevention and follow-up should be emphasized for these individuals, adequate to their neurological development, with prescription of artificial saliva when needed. When teeth are lost due to caries or congenitally absent, the utilization of total or partial dentures is indicated, and strict dental plaque control is fundamental to maintain the treatment and oral health of affected individuals [48, 58].

RAPP-HODGKIN SYNDROME

The Rapp-Hodgkin syndrome is a rare type of anhidrotic ectodermal dysplasia, with autosomal dominant inheritance [59, 60], and is characterized by cleft lip and palate, hypohidrosis, hypotrichosis (characterized by thin and sparse hair evolving to alopecia in adults) (Fig. **5.17**), absence of eyelashes and eyebrows, small mouth, narrow nose, hypospadia in males and nail dystrophy (Fig. **5.18**), abnormalities in the lacrimal ducts, auditory canals and ears, besides changes in tooth structures as oligodontia or anodontia (Fig. **5.19**) [61, 62]. There may be hyperthermia in early childhood. Individuals may also present short stature, maxillary hypoplasia, hearing loss, ptosis and depressed nasal bridge.

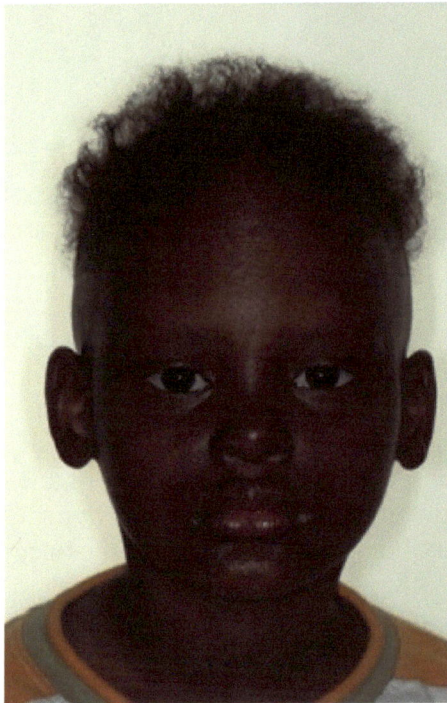

Fig. (5.17). Sparse hair, absent eyelashes and eyebrows in individual with Rapp-Hodgkin syndrome.

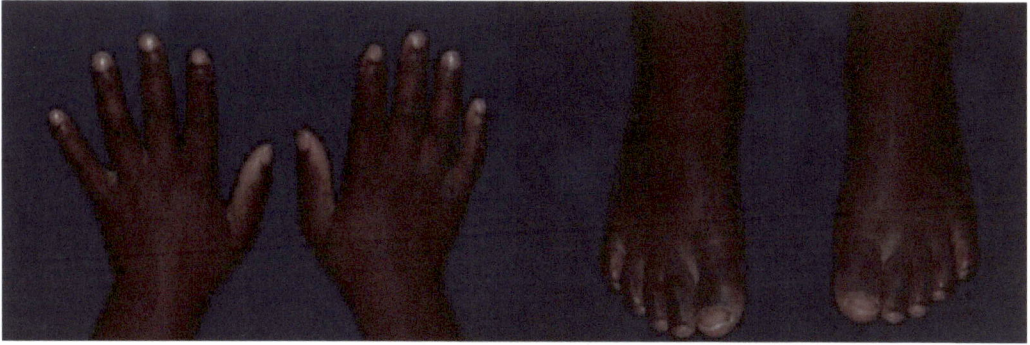

Fig. (5.18). Dry skin and nail dystrophy in the same individual with Rapp-Hodgkin syndrome presented in Fig. (**5.17**).

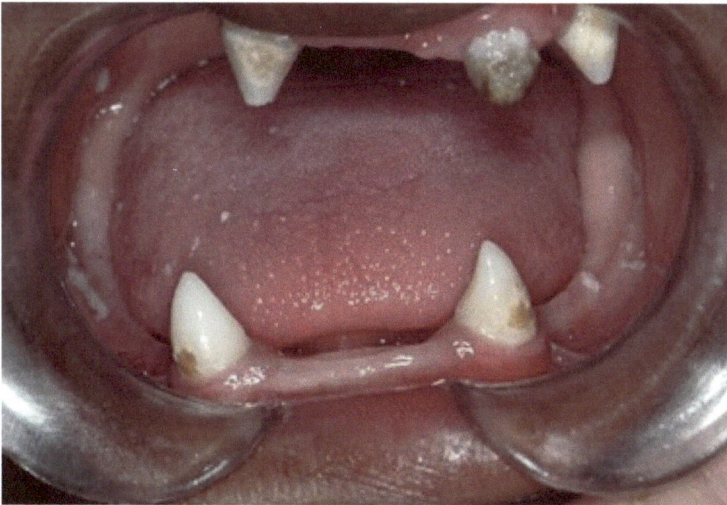

Fig. (5.19). Enamel hypoplasia and hypodontia of all molars and nearly all incisors in the same individual with Rapp-Hodgkin syndrome presented in Figs. (**5.17** and **5.18**).

It is believed that some cases may be incomplete manifestations of the EEC syndrome [21, 44]. Mutations in the TP63 gene have been reported in Rapp-Hodgkin syndrome [17, 49, 61, 63, 64]. The absence of ectrodactyly is an important signal for differential diagnosis with EEC syndrome.

The Rapp-Hodgkin syndrome is very similar to the AEC syndrome, being considered by some authors as varied expressions of the same disorder, when compared in relation to facial cleft and limb malformations [49, 65, 66].

The literature reports cases of oral manifestations including hypodontia, microdontia [61, 62, 67 - 69], tooth crown shape anomalies, delayed tooth eruption [69], unerupted premolars with good root formation, wide coronal pulp chamber (taurodontism), enamel hypoplasias [49], multiple caries, glossy tongue, besides congenital absence of the tongue frenum and sublingual caruncles [70]. These alterations increase the caries risk and impair the esthetics, which should be addressed in the dental management of individuals with Rapp-Hodgkin syndrome [59, 68, 69, 71, 72].

ROBIN SEQUENCE

The Robin sequence (RS) is classically described as a triad including micrognathia (Fig. **5.20**), glossoptosis and airway obstruction. Most cases (73-90%) are associated with U-shaped cleft palate [73] (Fig. **5.21**). Because of these characteristics, individuals with RS present respiratory and feeding difficulties, which are more frequent and severe in the neonatal period [74].

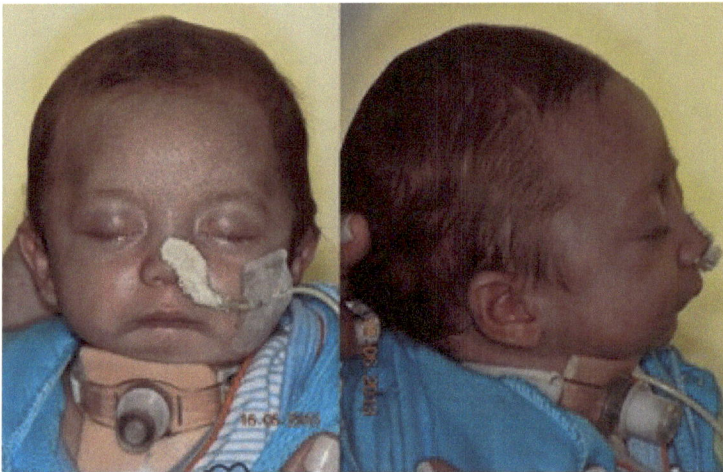

Fig. (5.20). Individual with Robin sequence. Notice the marked micrognathia, nasopharyngeal tube and tracheostomy.

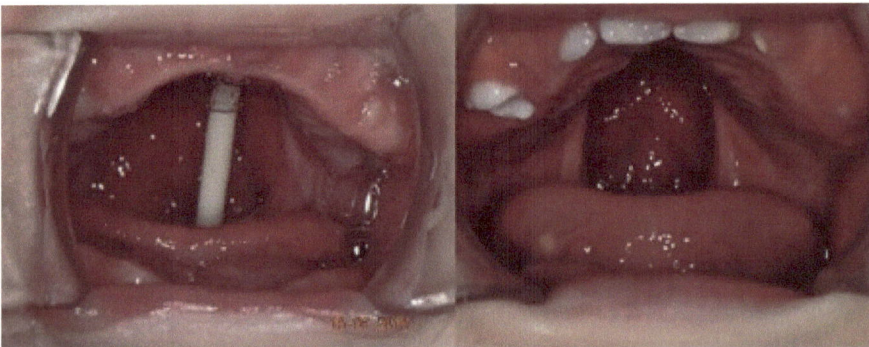

Fig. (5.21). Intraoral photographs of the same individual with Robin sequence presented in Fig. (**5.20**), at different ages. Notice the U-shaped cleft palate and the nasopharyngeal tube, placed for feeding.

The RS is not a syndrome, but rather a cascade of disorders, in which one anomaly causes the following. The mandible is small, leading to backward tongue positioning, which leads to airway obstruction.

The treatment options depend on the severity of airway obstruction. In case of mild airway obstruction, posture intervention (prone positioning) may be effective in up to 70% of cases [75]. The treatment options for severe cases include nasopharyngeal tube (Figs. **5.20** and **5.21**), mandibular distraction osteogenesis and tracheostomy (Fig. **5.20**) [76].

The estimated prevalence of Robin sequence is around 1/8,500 to 1/14,000 births [77 - 79], yet the achievement of more accurate data is impaired by the variability in diagnostic criteria [76].

This phenotype may be observed in isolation or combined with some syndromes [80]. The study of Izumi *et al.,* [81] observed 40% of cases of isolated RS and 60% associated with other syndromes, more commonly the Stickler and velocardiofacial syndromes.

The exact cause of Robin sequence is still unknown. The SOX9 gene, a critical chondrogenic regulator, has been associated with non-syndromic RS in families with more than one affected individual [82].

A recent study demonstrated that several non-codifying elements contribute to regulate the expression of the craniofacial gene SOX9; in RS, these craniofacial regulators are the site of deletions, contributing to the typical phenotype [83]. Jakobsen *et al.,* [84] investigated a series of unrelated individuals with RS and suggested that the etiology of non-syndromic RS is associated with lack of regulation of SOX9 and KCNJ2 genes, both in chromosome 17, one of which presented balanced translocation between chromosomes 2 and 17.

There are three main assumptions to explain the sequence of events in RS [76]: (a) hypoplastic mandible; (b) muscular and oropharyngeal deficiencies; (c) mandibular compression inside the womb. The theory of hypoplastic mandible is the main reported in the literature and has been demonstrated in animal models (especially in murines) [85]. It is believed that there is a primary defect in the Meckel cartilage, the embryonic structure involved in mandibular formation and growth. The mandibular hypoplasia would lead to small size of the oral cavity, abnormal tongue positioning and secondary impairment of palate closure [86].

In the hypothesis of muscular and oropharyngeal deficiency, it is believed that muscle hypotonia may lead to mandibular hypoplasia [76]. The persistence of feeding problems for weeks or months in children with RS whose respiratory problems were solved suggests abnormalities in pharyngeal mobility and tone. Fetal oral muscular activity, including swallowing, is also necessary for normal mandibular growth.

Finally, the theory of mandibular compression might be responsible for a small proportion of children with RS, especially in cases of pregnancy associated with fetal restriction as oligohydramnios or twin pregnancy. In fact, higher prevalence of twins has been reported in the population with RS compared to the general population [87, 88].

Concerning the orofacial characteristics, during the first months of life, the respiratory difficulties are naturally solved in many children with RS, thanks to the great increase in airway dimensions occurring in the first two years of life (3.5 times its original size) [89]. This improvement leads to a faster rate of mandibular growth, slower relative tongue growth and more anterior tongue positioning. Notwithstanding, normal mandibular arch dimensions are rarely attained in this population [89 - 91].

A cephalometric study analyzing the mandibular growth [90] revealed that individuals with RS present significantly smaller mandible compared to individuals with isolated cleft palate.

Individuals with RS present higher prevalence of hypodontia of permanent teeth, affecting nearly 30% to 50% [92, 93]. A recent study on individuals with non-syndromic RS demonstrated overall prevalence of hypodontia of permanent teeth of 32.9% (48 out of 146 individuals), with nearly two thirds presenting bilateral tooth agenesis. The most common pattern of hypodontia was the absence of both mandibular second premolars [94].

Individuals with RS present important clinical implications for dental treatment. Their neuropsychomotor development is usually normal, thus they may be able to comply with treatment. Attention should be given to individuals with respiratory difficulties who require restorative treatment in early ages, especially concerning the position of the dental chair (half-seated) and utilization of rubber dam, also with possibility of limited mouth opening. The indication for orthodontic/orthopedic treatment is restricted to individuals whose profile is not normalized during growth.

RICHIERI-COSTA-PEREIRA SYNDROME

The Richieri-Costa-Pereira syndrome (RCPS) was described in 1992, in Brazil, as a form of acrofacial dysostosis, presenting as main clinical manifestations the short stature, Robin sequence, mandibular cleft and pre- and postaxial anomalies of hands and clubfeet [95].

Later, other clinical signs of RCPS were reported in the literature including prominent and low-set ears (Fig. **5.22**), hypoplasia and proximal positioning of the thumbs, hypoplastic radius, clinodactyly of the fifth finger, radial deviation of the hands, hypoplastic first metacarpal bone and first phalanx [96, 97]; clavicular hypoplasia [97], mesomelic shortening of limbs; hypoplastic and short halluces (Fig. **5.23**) [34, 96], preaxial polydactyly of toes, and hypoplasia of radius, ulna, tibia and fibula [98].

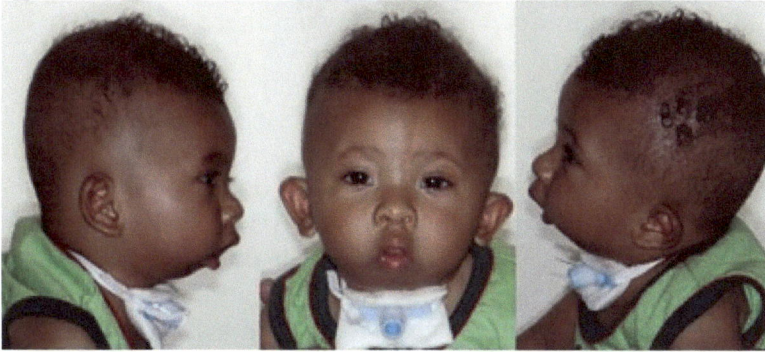

Fig. (5.22). Typical facial aspect in individual with Richieri-Costa-Pereira syndrome. Notice the prominent and low-set ears and marked micrognathia.

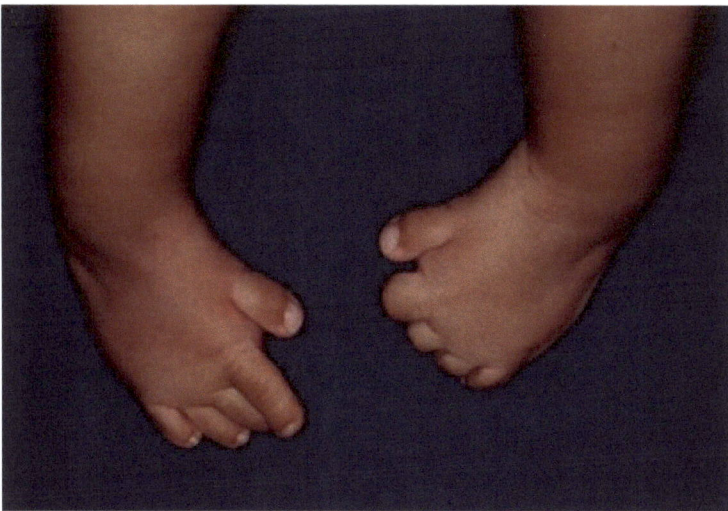

Fig. (5.23). Clubfeet and short halluces in the same individual with Richieri-Costa-Pereira syndrome presented in Fig. (**5.22**).

The presence of laryngeal malformations was described by Tabith Junior and Bento-Gonçalves [99, 100], including small or narrow larynx, absent or abnormal epiglottis and abnormal epiglottal folds. Consequently, the individuals present phonoarticulatory disorders as hoarse and blowy voice.

The neurological development in individuals with RCPS is considered normal [34, 95, 100 - 102], yet some studies demonstrated learning impairment, due to neuropsychological delay and language disturbances [96, 98].

An important characteristic in RCPS is the high frequency of airway obstruction and respiratory and feeding difficulties in the neonate [103], due to deficient growth of the head and neck region. Thus, these individuals require special support, especially in the first years of life, when there is greater risk of death [96].

The RCPS presents greater occurrence in female individuals (F:M=1.3:1) [96]. Concerning the etiology, the RCPS is a rare disorder of autosomal recessive inheritance. Only 33 cases have been reported so far, being 32 in Brazilian individuals [60, 104] and one French individual [105]. Even though most reports describe unrelated families, there is high prevalence of consanguineous marriages (44%) among non-syndromic parents of individuals with RCPS [96]. Also, most reported families are originated from a same restricted geographical area in Brazil (Vale do Ribeira region, state of São Paulo) [96]. Thus, a possibility has been raised of a common ancestor, yielding a founder effect of the syndrome [102].

Recently, a molecular biology study determined the genetic cause of RCPS, identifying a mutation present in two alleles of the EIF4A3 gene, located in chromosome 17q25, in 17 individuals. This alteration was characterized by excess repetition (14 to 16 copies) of one region rich in nitrogenous bases cytosine and guanine, which regulates functioning of the EIF4A3 gene. This gene is involved in the RNA metabolism, which participates in the morphogenesis of the mandible, larynx and limbs [104].

The orofacial aspects include retromicrognathia, microstomia, mandibular cleft involving the mandibular alveolar ridge (Fig. **5.24**), mandibular hypoplasia mandibular, high-arched palate and cleft palate. Also, the individuals present high prevalence of hypoplastic dental anomalies. Those more frequently found are hypodontia of mandibular incisors (due to the mandibular cleft) (Fig. **5.25**) and greater occurrence of hypodontia of the mandibular second premolars and demarcated creamy-white enamel opacities in maxillary premolars [106]. Cephalometric evaluation of individuals with RCPS compared with non-syndromic cases revealed statistically lower values for the SNB angle, maxillary and mandibular length, upper and lower anterior facial height and posterior facial height [107].

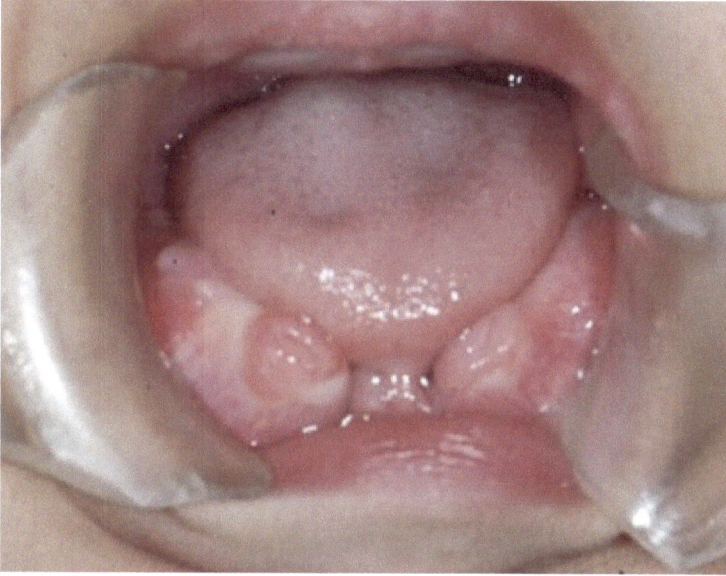

Fig. (5.24). Intraoral view of the same individual with Richieri-Costa-Pereira syndrome presented in Figs. (**5.22** and **5.23**). Notice the mandibular cleft.

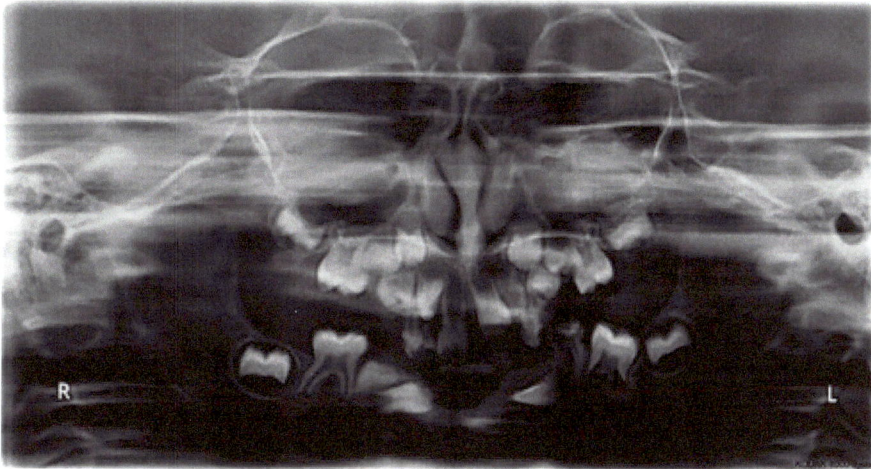

Fig. (5.25). Panoramic radiograph of the same individual with Richieri-Costa-Pereira syndrome presented in Figs. (**5.22** to **5.24**). Notice the bony aspect of the mandibular cleft and hypodontia of all mandibular incisors, mandibular left first and second premolars and mandibular right canine.

CONFLICT OF INTEREST

The author (editor) declares no conflict of interest, financial or otherwise.

ACKNOWLEDGEMENTS

Declared none.

REFERENCES

[1]   Jones KL, Adam MP. Evaluation and diagnosis of the dysmorphic infant. Clin Perinatol 2015; 42(2): 243-261, vii-viii.
        [http://dx.doi.org/10.1016/j.clp.2015.02.002] [PMID: 26042903]

[2]   Klein OD, Oberoi S, Huysseune A, Hovorakova M, Peterka M, Peterkova R. Developmental disorders of the dentition: an update. Am J Med Genet C Semin Med Genet 2013; 163C(4): 318-32.
        [http://dx.doi.org/10.1002/ajmg.c.31382] [PMID: 24124058]

[3]   Wallis D, Muenke M, Muenke M. Mutations in holoprosencephaly. Hum Mutat 2000; 16(2): 99-108.
        [http://dx.doi.org/10.1002/1098-1004(200008)16:2<99::AID-HUMU2>3.0.CO;2-0]   [PMID: 10923031]

[4]   Kauvar EF, Muenke M. Holoprosencephaly: recommendations for diagnosis and management. Curr Opin Pediatr 2010; 22(6): 687-95.
        [http://dx.doi.org/10.1097/MOP.0b013e32833f56d5] [PMID: 20859208]

[5]   Barr M Jr, Hanson JW, Currey K, *et al.* Holoprosencephaly in infants of diabetic mothers. J Pediatr 1983; 102(4): 565-8.
        [http://dx.doi.org/10.1016/S0022-3476(83)80185-1] [PMID: 6834191]

[6]   Miller EA, Rasmussen SA, Siega-Riz AM, Frías JL, Honein MA. Risk factors for non-syndromic holoprosencephaly in the National Birth Defects Prevention Study. Am J Med Genet C Semin Med Genet 2010; 154C(1): 62-72.
        [http://dx.doi.org/10.1002/ajmg.c.30244] [PMID: 20104597]

[7]   Johnson CY, Rasmussen SA. Non-genetic risk factors for holoprosencephaly. Am J Med Genet C Semin Med Genet 2010; 154C(1): 73-85.
        [http://dx.doi.org/10.1002/ajmg.c.30242] [PMID: 20104598]

[8]   McKusick VA. Holoprosencephaly 1; HPE1. Available at: http://omim.org/entry/236100

[9]   Becktor KB, Sverrild L, Pallisgaard C, Burhøj J, Kjaer I. Eruption of the central incisor, the intermaxillary suture, and maxillary growth in patients with a single median maxillary central incisor. Acta Odontol Scand 2001; 59(6): 361-6.
        [http://dx.doi.org/10.1080/000163501317153202] [PMID: 11831485]

[10]   Kjaer I, Becktor KB, Lisson J, Gormsen C, Russell BG. Face, palate, and craniofacial morphology in patients with a solitary median maxillary central incisor. Eur J Orthod 2001; 23(1): 63-73.
        [http://dx.doi.org/10.1093/ejo/23.1.63] [PMID: 11296511]

[11]   Nanni L, Ming JE, Du Y, *et al.* SHH mutation is associated with solitary median maxillary central incisor: a study of 13 patients and review of the literature. Am J Med Genet 2001; 102(1): 1-10.
        [http://dx.doi.org/10.1002/1096-8628(20010722)102:1<1::AID-AJMG1336>3.0.CO;2-U]   [PMID: 11471164]

[12]   McKusick VA. Solitary median maxillary central incisor; SMMCI. Available at: http://omim.org/entry/147250

[13]   McKusick VA. Van der Woude syndrome 1; VWS1. Available at: http://www.omim.org/entry/119300

[14]   Van Der Woude A. Fistula labii inferioris congenita and its association with cleft lip and palate. Am J Hum Genet 1954; 6(2): 244-56.
        [PMID: 13158329]

[15]   Rizos M, Spyropoulos MN. Van der Woude syndrome: a review. Cardinal signs, epidemiology, associated features, differential diagnosis, expressivity, genetic counselling and treatment. Eur J Orthod 2004; 26(1): 17-24.
        [http://dx.doi.org/10.1093/ejo/26.1.17] [PMID: 14994878]

[16]   Rintala AE, Ranta R. Lower lip sinuses: I. Epidemiology, microforms and transverse sulci. Br J Plast Surg 1981; 34(1): 26-30.
[http://dx.doi.org/10.1016/0007-1226(81)90090-4] [PMID: 7459520]

[17]   Celli J, Duijf P, Hamel BC, *et al.* Heterozygous germline mutations in the p53 homolog p63 are the cause of EEC syndrome. Cell 1999; 99(2): 143-53.
[http://dx.doi.org/10.1016/S0092-8674(00)81646-3] [PMID: 10535733]

[18]   Schutte BC, Bjork BC, Coppage KB, *et al.* A preliminary gene map for the Van der Woude syndrome critical region derived from 900 kb of genomic sequence at 1q32-q41. Genome Res 2000; 10(1): 81-94.
[PMID: 10645953]

[19]   Schinzel A, Kläusler M. The Van der Woude syndrome (dominantly inherited lip pits and clefts). J Med Genet 1986; 23(4): 291-4.
[http://dx.doi.org/10.1136/jmg.23.4.291] [PMID: 3746828]

[20]   King NM, Cheong CH, Sanares AM. Van der Woude syndrome: a report of two cases. J Clin Pediatr Dent 2004; 28(3): 267-71.
[http://dx.doi.org/10.17796/jcpd.28.3.t250869457555q58] [PMID: 15163158]

[21]   Gorlin RJ, Cohen MM Jr, Levin LS. Orofacial clefting syndromes: common and/or well-known syndromes. In: Gorlin RJ, Cohen MM, Hennekam RC, Eds. Syndromes of the head and neck New York. Oxford 1990; pp. 715-40.

[22]   Jobling R, Ferrier RA, McLeod R, Petrin AL, Murray JC, Thomas MA. Monozygotic twins with variable expression of Van der Woude syndrome. Am J Med Genet A 2011; 155A(8): 2008-10.
[http://dx.doi.org/10.1002/ajmg.a.34022] [PMID: 21739575]

[23]   Kondo S, Schutte BC, Richardson RJ, *et al.* Mutations in IRF6 cause Van der Woude and popliteal pterygium syndromes. Nat Genet 2002; 32(2): 285-9.
[http://dx.doi.org/10.1038/ng985] [PMID: 12219090]

[24]   Cervenka J, Gorlin RJ, Anderson VE. The syndrome of pits of the lower lip and cleft lip and/or palate. Genetic considerations. Am J Hum Genet 1967; 19(3 Pt 2): 416-32.
[PMID: 6026934]

[25]   Oberoi S, Vargervik K. Hypoplasia and hypodontia in Van der Woude syndrome. Cleft Palate Craniofac J 2005; 42(5): 459-66.
[http://dx.doi.org/10.1597/04-028.1] [PMID: 16149825]

[26]   Calzavara Pinton PG, Gavazzoni R, Carlino A, Leali C. [Van der Woude syndrome]. G Ital Dermatol Venereol 1989; 124(4): 171-3.
[PMID: 2807397]

[27]   Shprintzen RJ. Velo-cardio-facial syndrome: 30 Years of study. Dev Disabil Res Rev 2008; 14(1): 3-10.
[http://dx.doi.org/10.1002/ddrr.2] [PMID: 18636631]

[28]   Ryan AK, Goodship JA, Wilson DI, *et al.* Spectrum of clinical features associated with interstitial chromosome 22q11 deletions: a European collaborative study. J Med Genet 1997; 34(10): 798-804.
[http://dx.doi.org/10.1136/jmg.34.10.798] [PMID: 9350810]

[29]   da Silva Dalben G, Richieri-Costa A, de Assis Taveira LA. Tooth abnormalities and soft tissue changes in patients with velocardiofacial syndrome. Oral Surg Oral Med Oral Pathol Oral Radiol Endod 2008; 106(2): e46-51.
[http://dx.doi.org/10.1016/j.tripleo.2008.04.019] [PMID: 18554940]

[30]   Klingberg G, Hallberg U, Oskarsdóttir S. Oral health and 22q11 deletion syndrome: thoughts and experiences from the parents' perspectives. Int J Paediatr Dent 2010; 20(4): 283-92.
[http://dx.doi.org/10.1111/j.1365-263X.2010.01052.x] [PMID: 20536590]

[31]   Klingberg G, Lingström P, Oskarsdóttir S, Friman V, Bohman E, Carlén A. Caries-related saliva properties in individuals with 22q11 deletion syndrome. Oral Surg Oral Med Oral Pathol Oral Radiol Endod 2007; 103(4): 497-504.
[http://dx.doi.org/10.1016/j.tripleo.2006.09.018] [PMID: 17234437]

[32]   McKusick VA. Velocardiofacial syndrome. Available at: http://omim.org/entry/192430

[33]   Gurrieri F, Franco B, Toriello H, Neri G. Oral-facial-digital syndromes: review and diagnostic guidelines. Am J Med Genet A 2007; 143A(24): 3314-23.
[http://dx.doi.org/10.1002/ajmg.a.32032] [PMID: 17963220]

[34]   Graziadio C, Rosa RF, Zen PR, Flores JA, Paskulin GA. Richieri-Costa and Pereira form of acrofacial dysostosis: first description of an adult with mesomelic shortness of the lower limbs. Am J Med Genet A 2009; 149A(12): 2886-8.
[http://dx.doi.org/10.1002/ajmg.a.33109] [PMID: 19938093]

[35]   Azukizawa T, Yamamoto M, Narumiya S, Takano T. Oral-facial-digital syndrome type 1 with hypothalamic hamartoma and Dandy-Walker malformation. Pediatr Neurol 2013; 48(4): 329-32.
[http://dx.doi.org/10.1016/j.pediatrneurol.2012.12.016] [PMID: 23498571]

[36]   McKusick VA. Orofaciodigital syndrome I; OFD1. Available at: http://omim.org/entry/311200

[37]   Tagliani MM, Gomide MR, Carrara CF. Oral-facial-digital syndrome type 1: oral features in 12 patients submitted to clinical and radiographic examination. Cleft Palate Craniofac J 2010; 47(2): 162-6.
[http://dx.doi.org/10.1597/08-200.1] [PMID: 20210637]

[38]   Toriello HV. Heterogeneity and variability in the oral-facial-digital syndromes. Am J Med Genet Suppl 1988; 4 (Suppl.): 149-59.
[http://dx.doi.org/10.1002/ajmg.1320310515] [PMID: 3144982]

[39]   Toriello HV. Oral-facial-digital syndromes, 1992. Clin Dysmorphol 1993; 2(2): 95-105.
[http://dx.doi.org/10.1097/00019605-199304000-00001] [PMID: 8281288]

[40]   Thauvin-Robinet C, Cossée M, Cormier-Daire V, *et al.* Clinical, molecular, and genotype-phenotype correlation studies from 25 cases of oral-facial-digital syndrome type 1: a French and Belgian collaborative study. J Med Genet 2006; 43(1): 54-61.
[http://dx.doi.org/10.1136/jmg.2004.027672] [PMID: 16397067]

[41]   Dave KV, Patel SC, Dudhia BB, Panja P. Orofacial digital syndrome. Indian J Dent Res 2013; 24(1): 132-5.
[http://dx.doi.org/10.4103/0970-9290.114920] [PMID: 23852247]

[42]   Gunbay S, Zeytinoglu B, Ozkinay F, Ozkinay C, Oncag A. Orofaciodigital syndrome I: a case report. J Clin Pediatr Dent 1996; 20(4): 329-32.
[PMID: 9151628]

[43]   King NM, Sanares AM. Oral-facial-digital syndrome, Type I: a case report. J Clin Pediatr Dent 2002; 26(2): 211-5.
[http://dx.doi.org/10.17796/jcpd.26.2.d34417040174j35x] [PMID: 11878279]

[44]   McKusick VA. Ectrodactyly, ectodermal dysplasia, and cleft lip/palate syndrome 1; EEC1. Available at: http://omim.org/entry/129900

[45]   Koul M, Dwivedi R, Upadhyay V. Ectrodactyly-ectodermal dysplasia clefting syndrome (EEC syndrome). J Oral Biol Craniofac Res 2014; 4(2): 135-9.
[http://dx.doi.org/10.1016/j.jobcr.2014.08.002] [PMID: 25737931]

[46]   Alves LU, Pardono E, Otto PA, Mingroni Netto RC. A novel c.1037C > G (p.Ala346Gly) mutation in TP63 as cause of the ectrodactyly-ectodermal dysplasia and cleft lip/palate (EEC) syndrome. Genet Mol Biol 2015; 38(1): 37-41.
[http://dx.doi.org/10.1590/S1415-475738120140125] [PMID: 25983622]

[47]   Clements SE, Techanukul T, Coman D, Mellerio JE, McGrath JA. Molecular basis of EEC (ectrodactyly, ectodermal dysplasia, clefting) syndrome: five new mutations in the DNA-binding domain of the TP63 gene and genotype-phenotype correlation. Br J Dermatol 2010; 162(1): 201-7. [http://dx.doi.org/10.1111/j.1365-2133.2009.09496.x] [PMID: 19903181]

[48]   Sharma D, Kumar C, Bhalerao S, Pandita A, Shastri S, Sharma P. Ectrodactyly, ectodermal dysplasia, cleft lip and palate (EEC syndrome) with tetralogy of Fallot: a very rare combination. Front Pediatr 2015; 3: 51. [http://dx.doi.org/10.3389/fped.2015.00051] [PMID: 26137453]

[49]   van Straten C, Butow KW. Gene p63: In ectrodactyly-ectodermal dysplasia clefting, ankyloblepharon-ectodermal dysplasia, Rapp-Hodgkin syndrome. Ann Maxillofac Surg 2013; 3(1): 58-61. [http://dx.doi.org/10.4103/2231-0746.110085] [PMID: 23662261]

[50]   Iqbal Ali M, Aravinda K, Nigam NK, Ali I. Two interesting cases of EEC syndrome. J Oral Biol Craniofac Res 2013; 3(1): 45-8. [http://dx.doi.org/10.1016/j.jobcr.2013.02.001] [PMID: 25737881]

[51]   Celik TH, Buyukcam A, Simsek-Kiper PO, *et al.* A newborn with overlapping features of AEC and EEC syndromes. Am J Med Genet A 2011; 155A(12): 3100-3. [http://dx.doi.org/10.1002/ajmg.a.34328] [PMID: 22065614]

[52]   Rodini ES, Richieri-Costa A. EEC syndrome: report on 20 new patients, clinical and genetic considerations. Am J Med Genet 1990; 37(1): 42-53. [http://dx.doi.org/10.1002/ajmg.1320370112] [PMID: 2240042]

[53]   Shivaprakash PK, Joshi HV, Noorani H, Reddy V. Ectrodactyly, ectodermal dysplasia, and cleft lip/palate syndrome: A case report of "Incomplete syndrome". Contemp Clin Dent 2012; 3 (Suppl. 1): S115-7. [http://dx.doi.org/10.4103/0976-237X.95120] [PMID: 22629050]

[54]   Dhar RS, Bora A. Ectrodactyly-ectodermal dysplasia-cleft lip and palate syndrome. J Indian Soc Pedod Prev Dent 2014; 32(4): 346-9. [http://dx.doi.org/10.4103/0970-4388.140972] [PMID: 25231046]

[55]   Joseph R, Nath SG. Association of generalized aggressive periodontitis and ectrodactyly-ectodermal dysplasia-cleft syndrome. Indian J Hum Genet 2012; 18(2): 259-62. [http://dx.doi.org/10.4103/0971-6866.100793] [PMID: 23162310]

[56]   Tanboğa I, Pinçe S, Düzdar L. Dental management of a child with EEC syndrome. Int J Paediatr Dent 1992; 2(2): 99-103. [http://dx.doi.org/10.1111/j.1365-263X.1992.tb00017.x] [PMID: 1420102]

[57]   Ulukapi I, Bilgin T, Yalçin S. EEC syndrome (ectrodactyly-ectodermal dysplasia-clefting): a clinical case report. ASDC J Dent Child 2001; 68(5-6): 350-352, 302. [PMID: 11985198]

[58]   Pettit S, Campbell PR. Ectrodactyly-ectodermal dysplasia-clefting syndrome: the oral hygiene management of a patient with EEC. Spec Care Dentist 2010; 30(6): 250-4. [http://dx.doi.org/10.1111/j.1754-4505.2010.00162.x] [PMID: 21044105]

[59]   McKusick VA. Rapp-Hodgkin syndrome. Available at: http://omim.org/entry/129400

[60]   Rapp RS, Hodgkin WE. Anhidrotic ectodermal dysplasia: autosomal dominant inheritance with palate and lip anomalies. J Med Genet 1968; 5(4): 269-72. [http://dx.doi.org/10.1136/jmg.5.4.269] [PMID: 5713637]

[61]   Holder-Espinasse M, Abadie V, Cormier-Daire V, *et al.* Pierre Robin sequence: a series of 117 consecutive cases. J Pediatr 2001; 139(4): 588-90. [http://dx.doi.org/10.1067/mpd.2001.117784] [PMID: 11598609]

[62]   Moerman P, Fryns JP. Ectodermal dysplasia, Rapp-Hodgkin type in a mother and severe ectrodactyly-

ectodermal dysplasia-clefting syndrome (EEC) in her child. Am J Med Genet 1996; 63(3): 479-81.
[http://dx.doi.org/10.1002/(SICI)1096-8628(19960614)63:3<479::AID-AJMG12>3.0.CO;2-J] [PMID: 8737656]

[63] Bougeard G, Hadj-Rabia S, Faivre L, Sarafan-Vasseur N, Frébourg T. The Rapp-Hodgkin syndrome results from mutations of the TP63 gene. Eur J Hum Genet 2003; 11(9): 700-4.
[http://dx.doi.org/10.1038/sj.ejhg.5201004] [PMID: 12939657]

[64] Kantaputra PN, Hamada T, Kumchai T, McGrath JA. Heterozygous mutation in the SAM domain of p63 underlies Rapp-Hodgkin ectodermal dysplasia. J Dent Res 2003; 82(6): 433-7.
[http://dx.doi.org/10.1177/154405910308200606] [PMID: 12766194]

[65] Bertola DR, Kim CA, Albano LM, Scheffer H, Meijer R, van Bokhoven H. Molecular evidence that AEC syndrome and Rapp-Hodgkin syndrome are variable expression of a single genetic disorder. Clin Genet 2004; 66(1): 79-80.
[http://dx.doi.org/10.1111/j.0009-9163.2004.00278.x] [PMID: 15200513]

[66] Cambiaghi S, Tadini G, Barbareschi M, Menni S, Caputo R. Rapp-Hodgkin syndrome and AEC syndrome: are they the same entity? Br J Dermatol 1994; 130(1): 97-101.
[http://dx.doi.org/10.1111/j.1365-2133.1994.tb06891.x] [PMID: 8305327]

[67] Atasu M, Akesi S, Elçioglu N, Yatmaz PI, Ertas EB. A Rapp-Hodgkin like syndrome in three sibs: clinical, dental and dermatoglyphic study. Clin Dysmorphol 1999; 8(2): 101-10.
[PMID: 10319198]

[68] Dalben GdaS, Danelon LB, Carrara CF. Prosthetic rehabilitation of a child with Rapp-Hodgkin syndrome. J Dent Child (Chic) 2012; 79(2): 115-9.
[PMID: 22828770]

[69] Tosun G, Elbay U. Rapp-Hodgkin syndrome: clinical and dental findings. J Clin Pediatr Dent 2009; 34(1): 71-5.
[http://dx.doi.org/10.17796/jcpd.34.1.kr015833p1qg6873] [PMID: 19953814]

[70] Kantaputra PN, Pruksachatkunakorn C, Vanittanakom P. Rapp-Hodgkin syndrome with palmoplantar keratoderma, glossy tongue, congenital absence of lingual frenum and of sublingual caruncles: newly recognized findings. Am J Med Genet 1998; 79(5): 343-6.
[http://dx.doi.org/10.1002/(SICI)1096-8628(19981012)79:5<343::AID-AJMG3>3.0.CO;2-K] [PMID: 9779799]

[71] Crawford PJ, Aldred MJ, Clarke A, Tso MS. Rapp-Hodgkin syndrome: an ectodermal dysplasia involving the teeth, hair, nails, and palate. Report of a case and review of the literature. Oral Surg Oral Med Oral Pathol 1989; 67(1): 50-62.
[http://dx.doi.org/10.1016/0030-4220(89)90302-2] [PMID: 2643072]

[72] Schroeder HW Jr, Sybert VP. Rapp-Hodgkin ectodermal dysplasia. J Pediatr 1987; 110(1): 72-5.
[http://dx.doi.org/10.1016/S0022-3476(87)80291-3] [PMID: 3794888]

[73] Côté A, Fanous A, Almajed A, Lacroix Y. Pierre Robin sequence: review of diagnostic and treatment challenges. Int J Pediatr Otorhinolaryngol 2015; 79(4): 451-64.
[http://dx.doi.org/10.1016/j.ijporl.2015.01.035] [PMID: 25704848]

[74] Glynn F, Fitzgerald D, Earley MJ, Rowley H. Pierre Robin sequence: an institutional experience in the multidisciplinary management of airway, feeding and serous otitis media challenges. Int J Pediatr Otorhinolaryngol 2011; 75(9): 1152-5.
[http://dx.doi.org/10.1016/j.ijporl.2011.06.009] [PMID: 21764465]

[75] Mackay DR. Controversies in the diagnosis and management of the Robin sequence. J Craniofac Surg 2011; 22(2): 415-20.
[http://dx.doi.org/10.1097/SCS.0b013e3182074799] [PMID: 21403570]

[76] Tan TY, Kilpatrick N, Farlie PG. Developmental and genetic perspectives on Pierre Robin sequence. Am J Med Genet C Semin Med Genet 2013; 163C(4): 295-305.

[http://dx.doi.org/10.1002/ajmg.c.31374] [PMID: 24127256]

[77]   Bush PG, Williams AJ. Incidence of the Robin Anomalad (Pierre Robin syndrome). Br J Plast Surg
       1983; 36(4): 434-7.
       [http://dx.doi.org/10.1016/0007-1226(83)90123-6] [PMID: 6626822]

[78]   Printzlau A, Andersen M. Pierre Robin sequence in Denmark: a retrospective population-based
       epidemiological study. Cleft Palate Craniofac J 2004; 41(1): 47-52.
       [http://dx.doi.org/10.1597/02-055] [PMID: 14697070]

[79]   van den Elzen AP, Semmekrot BA, Bongers EM, Huygen PL, Marres HA. Diagnosis and treatment of
       the Pierre Robin sequence: results of a retrospective clinical study and review of the literature. Eur J
       Pediatr 2001; 160(1): 47-53.
       [http://dx.doi.org/10.1007/s004310000646] [PMID: 11195018]

[80]   McKusick VA. Robin sequence with cleft mandible and limb anomalies. Available at:
       http://www.omim.org/entry/268305

[81]   Izumi K, Konczal LL, Mitchell AL, Jones MC. Underlying genetic diagnosis of Pierre Robin
       sequence: retrospective chart review at two children's hospitals and a systematic literature review. J
       Pediatr 2012; 160(4): 645-650.e2.
       [http://dx.doi.org/10.1016/j.jpeds.2011.09.021] [PMID: 22048048]

[82]   Benko S, Fantes JA, Amiel J, *et al*. Highly conserved non-coding elements on either side of SOX9
       associated with Pierre Robin sequence. Nat Genet 2009; 41(3): 359-64.
       [http://dx.doi.org/10.1038/ng.329] [PMID: 19234473]

[83]   Gordon CT, Attanasio C, Bhatia S, *et al*. Identification of novel craniofacial regulatory domains
       located far upstream of SOX9 and disrupted in Pierre Robin sequence. Hum Mutat 2014; 35(8): 1011-
       20.
       [http://dx.doi.org/10.1002/humu.22606] [PMID: 24934569]

[84]   Jakobsen LP, Ullmann R, Christensen SB, *et al*. Pierre Robin sequence may be caused by
       dysregulation of SOX9 and KCNJ2. J Med Genet 2007; 44(6): 381-6.
       [http://dx.doi.org/10.1136/jmg.2006.046177] [PMID: 17551083]

[85]   Schubert J, Jahn H, Berginski M. Experimental aspects of the pathogenesis of Robin sequence. Cleft
       Palate Craniofac J 2005; 42(4): 372-6.
       [http://dx.doi.org/10.1597/03-166.1] [PMID: 16001918]

[86]   Hanson JW, Smith DW. U-shaped palatal defect in the Robin anomalad: developmental and clinical
       relevance. J Pediatr 1975; 87(1): 30-3.
       [http://dx.doi.org/10.1016/S0022-3476(75)80063-1] [PMID: 1151545]

[87]   Holder-Espinasse M, Martin-Coignard D, Escande F, Manouvrier-Hanu S. A new mutation in TP63 is
       associated with age-related pathology. Eur J Hum Genet 2007; 15(11): 1115-20.
       [http://dx.doi.org/10.1038/sj.ejhg.5201888] [PMID: 17609671]

[88]   Knottnerus AC, de Jong DJ, Haumann TJ, Mulder JW. Higher incidence of twins in infants with Pierre
       Robin sequence. Cleft Palate Craniofac J 2001; 38(3): 284.
       [http://dx.doi.org/10.1597/1545-1569(2001)038<0285:LTTE>2.0.CO;2] [PMID: 11386439]

[89]   Figueroa AA, Glupker TJ, Fitz MG, BeGole EA. Mandible, tongue, and airway in Pierre Robin
       sequence: a longitudinal cephalometric study. Cleft Palate Craniofac J 1991; 28(4): 425-34.
       [http://dx.doi.org/10.1597/1545-1569(1991)028<0425:MTAAIP>2.3.CO;2] [PMID: 1742314]

[90]   Daskalogiannakis J, Ross RB, Tompson BD. The mandibular catch-up growth controversy in Pierre
       Robin sequence. Am J Orthod Dentofacial Orthop 2001; 120(3): 280-5.
       [http://dx.doi.org/10.1067/mod.2001.115038] [PMID: 11552127]

[91]   Staudt CB, Gnoinski WM, Peltomäki T. Upper airway changes in Pierre Robin sequence from
       childhood to adulthood. Orthod Craniofac Res 2013; 16(4): 202-13.
       [PMID: 23350818]

[92] Andersson E-M, Sandvik L, Abyholm F, Semb G. Clefts of the secondary palate referred to the Oslo Cleft Team: epidemiology and cleft severity in 994 individuals. Cleft Palate Craniofac J 2010; 47(4): 335-42.
[http://dx.doi.org/10.1597/07-230.1] [PMID: 19860491]

[93] Ranta R, Rintala AE. The Pierre Robin anomalad--comparisons of some disturbances in the formation of the teeth and the lower lip. Proc Finn Dent Soc 1983; 79(4): 155-61.
[PMID: 6664980]

[94] Antonarakis GS, Suri S. Prevalence and patterns of permanent tooth agenesis in patients with nonsyndromic Pierre Robin sequence. Am J Orthod Dentofac Orthop 2014; 145: 452-60.

[95] Richieri-Costa A, Pereira SC. Short stature, Robin sequence, cleft mandible, pre/postaxial hand anomalies, and clubfoot: a new autosomal recessive syndrome. Am J Med Genet 1992; 42(5): 681-7.
[http://dx.doi.org/10.1002/ajmg.1320420511] [PMID: 1632438]

[96] Favaro FP, Zechi-Ceide RM, Alvarez CW, et al. Richieri-Costa-Pereira syndrome: a unique acrofacial dysostosis type. An overview of the Brazilian cases. Am J Med Genet A 2011; 155A(2): 322-31.
[http://dx.doi.org/10.1002/ajmg.a.33806] [PMID: 21271648]

[97] Golbert MB, Dewes LO, Philipsen VR, Wachholz RS, Deutschendorf C, Leite JC. New clinical findings in the Richieri-Costa/Pereira type of acrofacial dysostosis. Clin Dysmorphol 2007; 16(2): 85-8.
[http://dx.doi.org/10.1097/MCD.0b013e3280464ff6] [PMID: 17351350]

[98] Guion-Almeida ML, Richieri-Costa A. Autosomal recessive short stature, Robin sequence, cleft mandible, pre/postaxial limb anomalies, and clubfeet: report of a patient with polydactyly of the halluces. Braz J Dysmorphol Speech Hear Disord 1998; 2: 27-30.

[99] Tabith A Jr, Bento-Gonçalves CG. Laryngeal malformation in the Richieri-Costa-Pereira acrofacial dysostosis: description of two new patients. Am J Med Genet A 2003; 122A(2): 133-8.
[http://dx.doi.org/10.1002/ajmg.a.10227] [PMID: 12955765]

[100] Tabith Júnior A, Gonçalves CG. Laryngeal malformations in the Richieri-Costa and Pereira form of acrofacial dysostosis. Am J Med Genet 1996; 66(4): 399-402.
[http://dx.doi.org/10.1002/(SICI)1096-8628(19961230)66:4<399::AID-AJMG3>3.0.CO;2-G] [PMID: 8989456]

[101] Richieri-Costa A, Brandão-Almeida IL. Short stature, Robin sequence, cleft mandible, pre/postaxial hand anomalies, and clubfoot: another affected Brazilian patient born to consanguineous parents. Am J Med Genet 1997; 71(2): 233-5.
[http://dx.doi.org/10.1002/(SICI)1096-8628(19970808)71:2<233::AID-AJMG23>3.0.CO;2-E] [PMID: 9217230]

[102] Richieri-Costa A, Pereira SC. Autosomal recessive short stature, Robin sequence, cleft mandible, pre/postaxial hand anomalies, and clubfeet in male patients. Am J Med Genet 1993; 47(5): 707-9.
[http://dx.doi.org/10.1002/ajmg.1320470524] [PMID: 8267000]

[103] Wagener S, Rayatt SS, Tatman AJ, Gornall P, Slator R. Management of infants with Pierre Robin sequence. Cleft Palate Craniofac J 2003; 40(2): 180-5.
[http://dx.doi.org/10.1597/1545-1569(2003)040<0180:MOIWPR>2.0.CO;2] [PMID: 12605525]

[104] Favaro FP, Alvizi L, Zechi-Ceide RM, et al. A noncoding expansion in EIF4A3 causes Richieri-Costa-Pereira syndrome, a craniofacial disorder associated with limb defects. Am J Hum Genet 2014; 94(1): 120-8.
[http://dx.doi.org/10.1016/j.ajhg.2013.11.020] [PMID: 24360810]

[105]　Walter-Nicolet E, Coëslier A, Joriot S, Kacet N, Moerman A, Manouvrier-Hanu S. The Richieri-Costa and Pereira form of acrofacial dysostosis: first case in a non-Brazilian infant. Am J Med Genet 1999; 87(5): 430-3.
[http://dx.doi.org/10.1002/(SICI)1096-8628(19991222)87:5<430::AID-AJMG11>3.0.CO;2-9] [PMID: 10594883]

[106]　Severini JM, da Silva Dalben G, Richieri-Costa A, Ozawa TO. Dental anomalies in Richieri-Costa-Pereira syndrome. Oral Surg Oral Med Oral Pathol Oral Radiol 2012; 114(1): 99-106.
[http://dx.doi.org/10.1016/j.oooo.2012.03.009] [PMID: 22727098]

[107]　Pita Pardo MD. Relações maxilomandibulares na Sindrome de Richieri-Costa-Pereira. Bauru 2013. monograph

CHAPTER 6

Craniosynostosis Syndromes

Ana Lúcia Pompéia Fraga de Almeida[*] and **Gisele da Silva Dalben**[*]

Bauru School of Dentistry and Hospital for Rehabilitation of Craniofacial Anomalies, University of São Paulo, Brazil

Abstract: Craniosynostosis is the premature fusion of cranial sutures. This chapter addresses the craniosynostosis syndromes, which involve this premature fusion of cranial sutures associated with important disorders to the craniofacial complex and teeth, requiring emphasis on prevention, special care during dental treatment, and a multidisciplinary team approach for their full rehabilitation from early infancy through adulthood.

Keywords: Acrocephalosyndactylia, Acrocephalosyndactyly type II, Craniosynostoses, Craniofacial dysostosis, Dental care, Jackson-Weiss syndrome, Kaplan Plauchu Fitch syndrome, Multiple congenital anomalies syndrome with cloverleaf skull, Pfeiffer type acrocephalosyndactyly, Saethre-Chotzen syndrome with eyelid anomalies, Shprintzen Goldberg craniosynostosis, Tooth abnormalities.

Craniosynostosis, or craniostenosis, is a congenital disorder that causes premature closure of cranial sutures [1, 2], caused by mutations in genes CDC45, TWIST1, TCF12, and others, with an important role in cell division. In normal conditions, at birth, the child presents separated cranial bones, yet firmly connected to each other by fibrous structures called sutures. On the margins of these sutures there is intense metabolic activity with bone formation, which is involved with cranial growth. The cranial growth is directly proportional to brain growth and is very marked in the first two years of life. The premature closure of one or several cranial sutures reduces its bone synthesis activity, causing craniofacial deformities.

[*] **Corresponding author Ana Lúcia Pompéia Fraga de Almeida:** Bauru School of Dentistry and Hospital for Rehabilitation of Craniofacial Anomalies, University of São Paulo, Bauru, Brazil; Tel/Fax: +55 14 3235-8000; E-mail: analmeida@usp.br
[*] **Gisele da Silva Dalben:** Hospital for Rehabilitation of Craniofacial Anomalies, University of São Paulo, Bauru, Brazil; Tel/Fax: +55 14 3235-8000; E-mail: gsdalben@usp.br

In single suture craniosynostosis the cranial deformities are predictable, and the affected suture may be inferred from the cranial shape. Some descriptive denominations of cranial shape are related to the involvement of certain cranial sutures, as follows: scaphocephaly, for sagittal suture craniosynostosis (between the parietal bones), trigonocephaly for the metopic suture (between the fetal frontal bones), anterior plagiocephaly for the coronal suture (between frontal and parietal bones) unilaterally, brachycephaly for the coronal suture bilaterally, and posterior plagiocephaly for the lambdoid suture (between occipital and parietal bones) unilaterally [2, 3].

The craniosynostoses may be classified, according to the number of affected sutures, as simple or multiple; according to the etiology, as primary or of unknown cause, and secondary or of known cause; and according to the association with other malformations, as non-syndromic and syndromic. These classifications are not mutually excluding. The most frequent craniosynostoses are simple, primary and non-syndromic. The syndromes more frequently associated with craniosynostoses are the Apert and Crouzon syndromes, which are usually hereditary. With rare exceptions, the diagnosis of craniosynostoses is established at birth. Besides cranial deformities, the craniosynostoses may cause neurological problems due to the restrictive effect on brain growth if not treated timely, especially in multiple and syndromic craniosynostoses. The diagnosis of craniosynostoses may be suspected by analysis of the cranial shape and confirmed by radiography, computed tomography and magnetic resonance imaging.

The treatment of craniosynostoses is fundamentally surgical. Its correction aims at esthetic improvement and prevention of occasional neurological disorders. Usually, craniosynostoses should be corrected before 6 months of age [4].

APERT SYNDROME

The first description of Apert syndrome, or acrocephalosyndactyly, is assigned to Apert [5], yet it had been previously described by Wheaton in 1894 [6]. It is an autosomal dominant disorder assigned to mutations in the FGFR 2 gene in chromosome 10q26. The estimated prevalence ranges from 1 in 65,000 to 160,000 births to 1 in each 2 millions in the general population due to the high neonatal mortality, especially when craniosynostosis is not treated timely [6 - 8]. It may be diagnosed prenatally by ultrasound examination.

It is characterized by craniosynostosis of the coronal sutures. The face is typical with broad and high forehead, hyperteleorbitism, shallow orbits, proptosis and downslanting palpebral fissures (Fig. **6.1**). The nasal bridge is depressed and there may be choanal stenosis or atresia. The palate is narrow, with possibility of cleft palate and bifid uvula [9, 10]; however, the presence of marked hyperplasia of the palatal mucosa may lead to a mistaken diagnosis of cleft palate (Fig. **6.2**). Individuals with this syndrome may present cardiovascular alterations; genitourinary disorders with hydronephrosis, cryptorchidism and vaginal atresia; and abdominal disturbances including esophageal atresia and ectopic anus. It is differentiated from other multiple craniosynostosis syndromes by the presence of symmetric severe syndactyly on the hands and feet, involving soft or hard and soft tissues, usually affecting the second, third and fourth digits with a single nail (Figs. **6.3** and **6.4**) [9]. There seems to be alterations in the anterior cranial base cartilage at onset of intrauterine life, with compensatory alterations in cranial development at the onset of postnatal life [6 - 8].

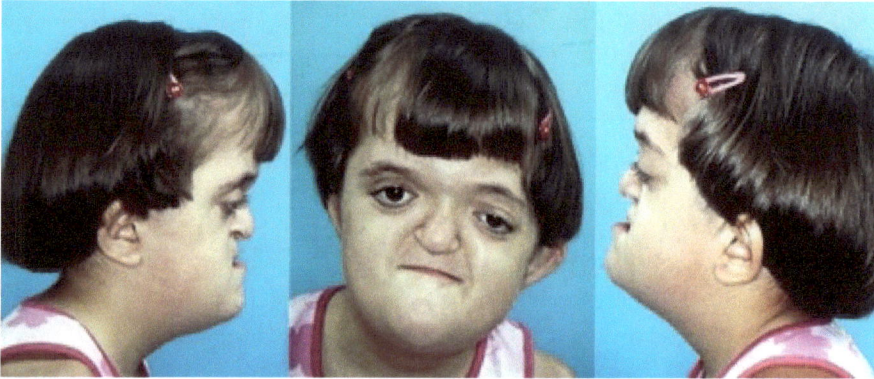

Fig. (6.1). Characteristic facial aspect in Apert syndrome. Notice the high and broad forehead, depressed nasal bridge, proptosis, and Class III facial pattern.

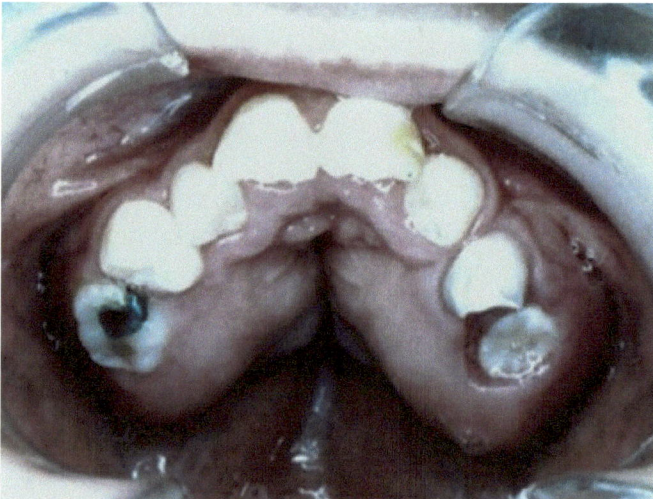

Fig. (6.2). Characteristic marked hyperplasia of the palatal mucosa in the same individual with Apert syndrome shown in Fig. (**6.1**).

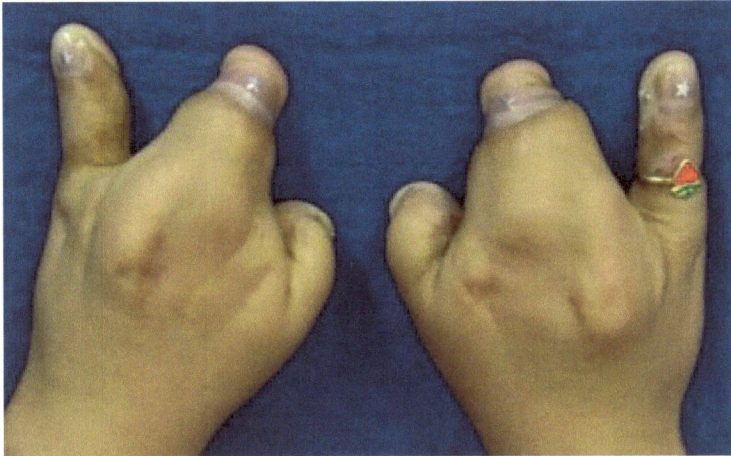

Fig. (6.3). Syndactyly affecting the second, third and fourth digits in the same individual with Apert syndrome shown in Figs. (**6.1** and **6.2**).

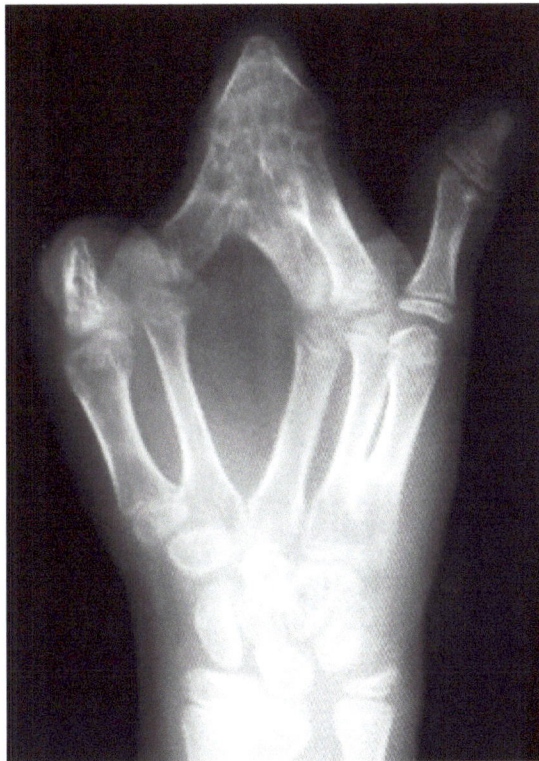

Fig. (6.4). Radiographic aspect of syndactyly affecting the hard tissues in the same individual presented in Figs. (**6.1** to **6.3**).

Intellectual development is usually normal, yet there may be intellectual disability in case of increased intracranial pressure due to lack of timely management of the craniosynostosis [11]. The intelligence also seems to be related with socioeconomic status of the family [12].

Most cases are sporadic and represent new mutations. There are reports of association with older paternal age [6]. Despite the autosomal dominant inheritance, the recurrence is low, possibly due to the low rate of reproduction of these individuals [13].

The several descriptions of oral features in individuals with Apert syndrome include the high-arched and deformed palate [9, 13, 14], eruption disturbances, gingival hypertrophy (which may also complicate tooth eruption), multiple hypodontia (Fig. **6.5**) [9, 14 - 16], eruption delay, which is more marked in older individuals [17], ectopic eruption (Fig. **6.6**) [14, 15, 18], and paddle-shaped incisors [15]. From an orthodontic standpoint, there is mouth breathing, Class III malocclusion (Figs. **6.7** and **6.8**), maxillary hypoplasia and retropositioning, relative mandibular prognathism, reduced mandibular ramus and body, backward mandibular rotation, buccal tipping of maxillary incisors, lingual tipping of mandibular incisors, anterior open bite and posterior crossbite, negative overjet and overbite, increased lower anterior facial height and reduced upper anterior facial height, high-arched palate and tooth crowding in both dental arches (Figs. **6.2** and **6.6**) [9, 15, 18 - 20]. Other authors reported greater dimension of the mandibular ramus and smaller mandibular body with normal gonial angle [21].

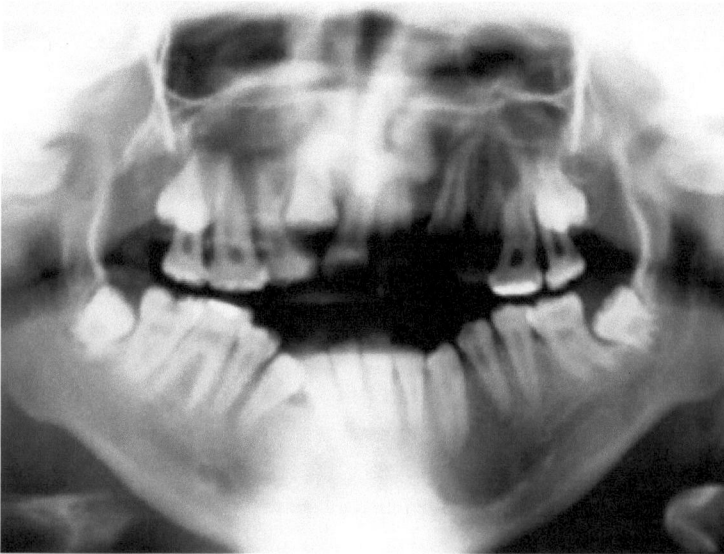

Fig. (6.5). Hypodontia of maxillary right and left lateral incisors, maxillary right canine, maxillary left first premolar and mandibular right canine in individual with Apert syndrome.

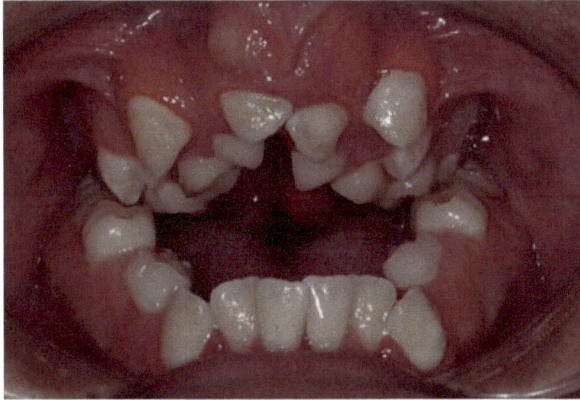

Fig. (6.6). Ectopic eruption of several teeth due to space restraint in individual with Apert syndrome.

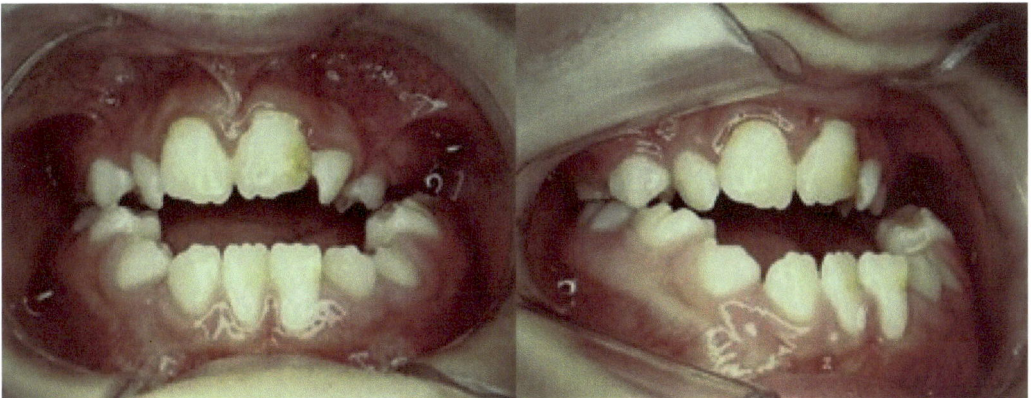

Fig. (6.7). Anterior open bite, posterior crossbite and Class III malocclusion in individual with Apert syndrome.

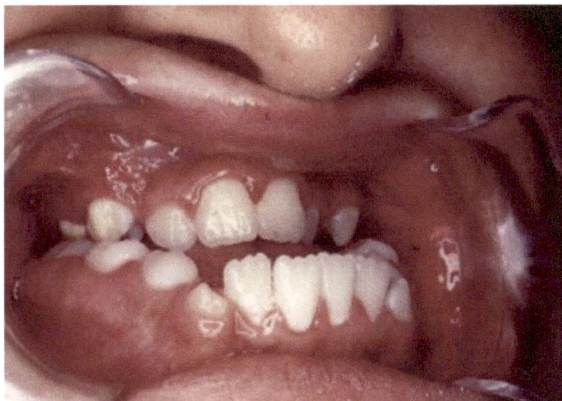

Fig. (6.8). Severe Class III malocclusion in individual with Apert syndrome.

With regard to the oral health of affected individuals, there are reports of high caries prevalence with early tooth loss (Fig. **6.9**) and difficult oral hygiene control due to malformation of the hands [20, 22] (Fig. **6.10**). The most thorough study about the oral health of these individuals was conducted by Mustafa *et al.* [4] on 57 children with craniosynostosis (11 with Apert, 21 Crouzon, 5 Pfeiffer, 3 Saethre-Chotzen syndromes, and 17 non-syndromic cases) aged 3 to 16 years, compared to a control group matched for gender, age and ethnicity. Higher frequency of caries was observed for the study group, yet with higher dmft index for the control group, which the authors assigned to the fact that children in the study group attended a multidisciplinary clinic since early childhood. The study group exhibited greater frequency of gingivitis in the permanent teeth, and both groups exhibited similar results concerning the presence of enamel defects and microbiological analysis. The study group presented greater amount of dental plaque, probably because oral hygiene is impaired by the presence of tooth crowding, evidencing the need of regular professional prophylaxis.

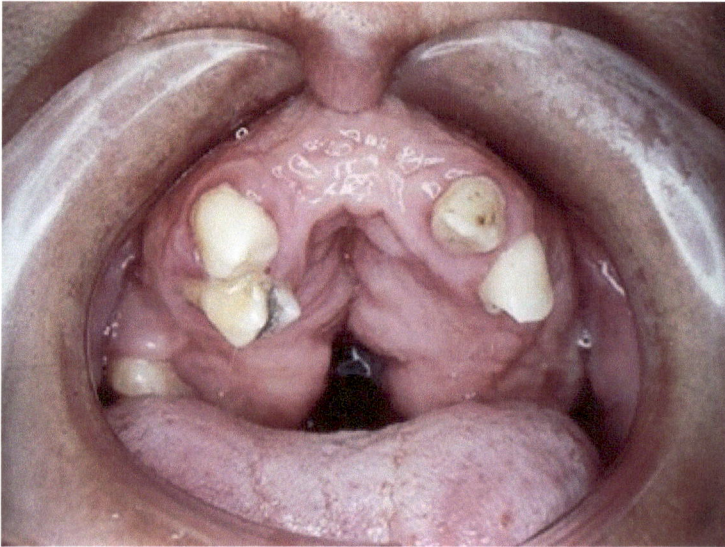

Fig. (6.9). Extensive tooth loss and poor oral health in individual with Apert syndrome.

Syndactyly of the hands is one of the main characteristics of these individuals. For this reason, electric toothbrushes (Fig. **6.10**) provide greater comfort and safety during toothbrushing, thanks to their rounded shape and large handle diameter. Additionally, these individuals seem to prefer the utilization of electric toothbrushes because they do not require complex movements for dental plaque removal.

The oral hygiene control of affected individuals may also be impaired by the presence of enamel defects, including hypoplasias and enamel opacities (Fig.

6.11) [14]. Alike the aforementioned report of Mustafa *et al.* [4], Dalben *et al.* [22] also observed high amount of dental plaque and poor oral hygiene control in individuals with Apert syndrome, yet similar findings were also observed for individuals with Crouzon syndrome, described below in this chapter, who do not have malformations of the hands. Thus, it might be inferred that other factors related to both syndromes, such as tooth crowding and abnormal maxillomandibular relationships, may significantly impair the oral hygiene control.

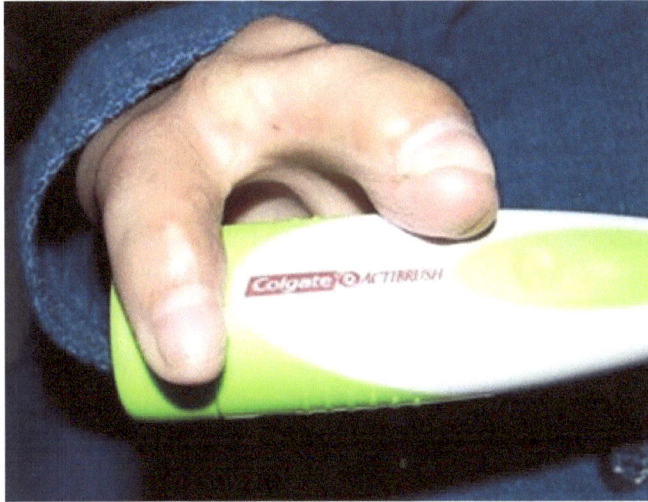

Fig. (6.10). Individual with Apert syndrome and severe malformation of the hand holding an electric toothbrush.

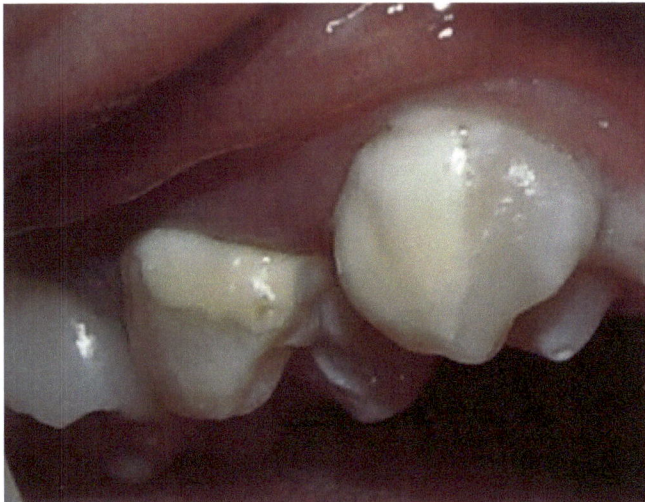

Fig. (6.11). Enamel opacities in individual with Apert syndrome.

Comparison of craniofacial features between Apert and Crouzon syndromes evidences the presence of smaller mandibular body and ramus and greater gonial angle for the Crouzon syndrome [21]. It is reported that individuals with Apert syndrome present greater frequency and severity of high-arched palate, anterior open bite, midline deviation, crowding of maxillary teeth and facial shortening compared to the Crouzon syndrome [9, 15, 23]. There are also reports of more severe maxillary deficiency, inadequate interincisor relationship and retrusion of the soft tissue profile in Apert syndrome, which are more marked in childhood, with greater similarity between these with over age [24].

Dental care in individuals with Apert syndrome mainly requires dental plaque control and counseling for caretakers concerning oral hygiene at home, due to the usual difficulty of these individuals to perform oral hygiene by themselves, because of syndactyly and severe tooth crowding [9]. Despite the low caries prevalence, the plaque index is usually high, as well as the frequency of gingivitis, and regular follow-up with professional prophylaxis is recommended. Compliance is usually good, since most affected individuals do not present neurological disorders [11, 12]. From an orthodontic standpoint, many individuals require distraction osteogenesis or orthognathic surgery, due to maxillary deficiency. Maxillary advancement may be helpful to reduce the exophthalmos, thanks to advancement of the lower rim of the orbit, which is shallow in these individuals. Please refer to Chapter 9 for further information on the surgical-orthodontic management of individuals with Apert syndrome.

Oral hygiene instruction, professional prophylaxis and orthodontic treatment for alignment of malpositioned or crowded teeth improve the oral hygiene conditions and consequently reduce the risk of caries and gingivitis [9, 25].

CROUZON SYNDROME

The Crouzon syndrome, or craniofacial dysostosis, is an autosomal dominant disorder related to mutations in the FGFR 2 gene on chromosome 10q26. Its familial occurrence was observed by Crouzon [26], who described the syndrome. It is characterized by craniosynostosis of the coronal, sagittal and lambdoid sutures with brachycephaly, prominent forehead, maxillary hypoplasia, shallow orbits, significant orbital proptosis and optical atrophy, with possibility of conjunctivitis due to exposure of the conjunctiva and visual impairment (Fig. **6.12**). Individuals present a beak-shaped nose. Alike the Apert syndrome, there is hyperplasia of the palatal mucosa (Fig. **6.13**) and etiological association with increasing paternal age, yet without limb malformations. There may be calcification of the stylohyoid ligament. The primary abnormality in this syndrome seems to be the fusion of bone sutures and synchondroses during late fetal life or early childhood [6, 8, 27]. Occasionally there may be intellectual impairment, possibly associated with the increased intracranial pressure [11].

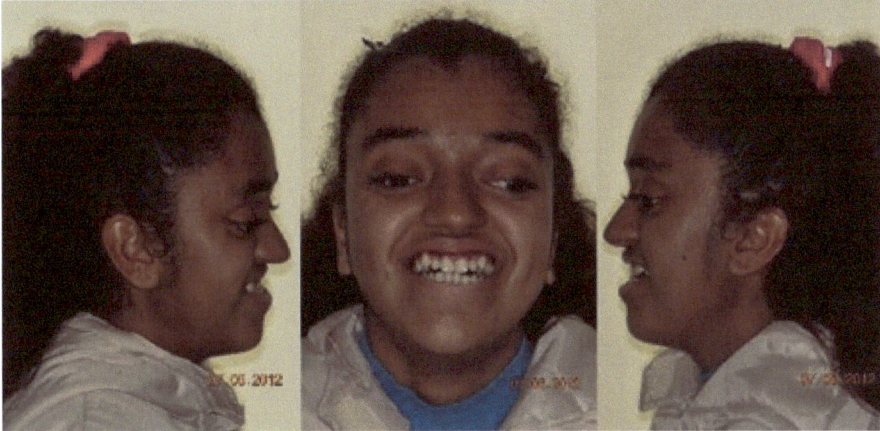

Fig. (6.12). Characteristic facial aspect in Crouzon syndrome. Notice the proptosis, beak-shaped nose and Class III facial pattern.

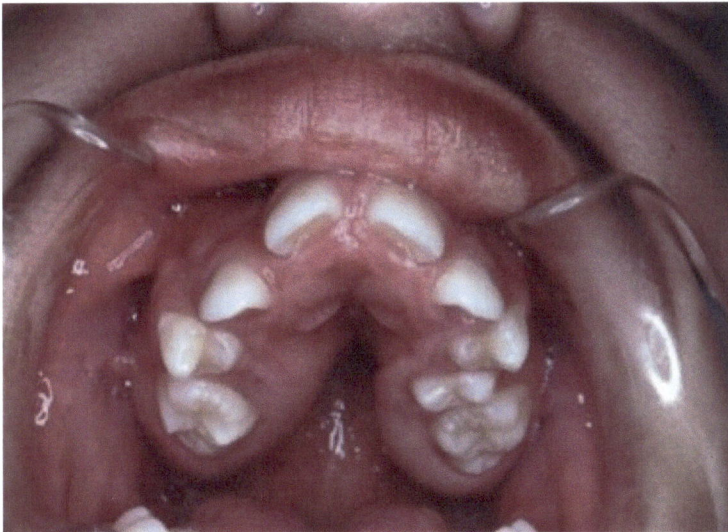

Fig. (6.13). Characteristic marked hyperplasia of the palatal mucosa in an individual with Crouzon syndrome.

A thorough study about the oral health status of individuals with craniosynostosis was conducted by Mustafa *et al.* [4] (please refer to the Apert syndrome section). The characteristic oral features of Crouzon syndrome include reduced maxillary length with nearly normal width and increased height, counterclockwise maxillary rotation, reduced SNA angle, short maxillary arch, deficiency vertical and horizontal growth of the middle facial third, mandibular prognathism with normal mandibular growth, smaller mandibular body, greater or closed gonial angle, narrow or increased mandibular ramus (Fig. **6.14**), Angle Class III malocclusion (Fig. **6.15**), anterior open bite (Fig. **6.14**), reports of good intra-arch relationship and greater dimension of the mandibular ramus [21, 28 - 30].

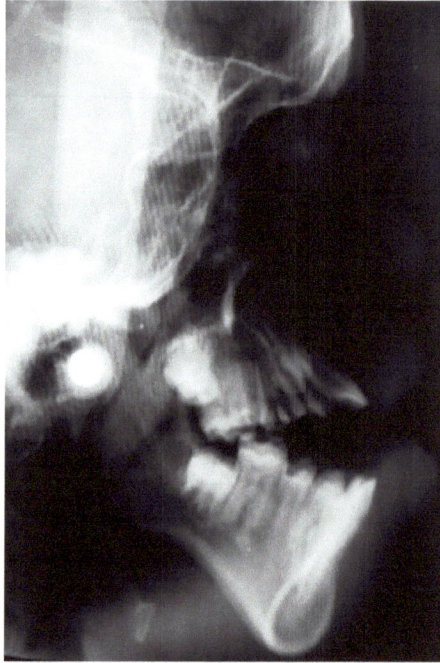

Fig. (6.14). Lateral cephalogram of individual with Crouzon syndrome with severe Angle Class III malocclusion. Notice the increased gonial angle, Angle Class III relationship and severe skeletal anterior open bite.

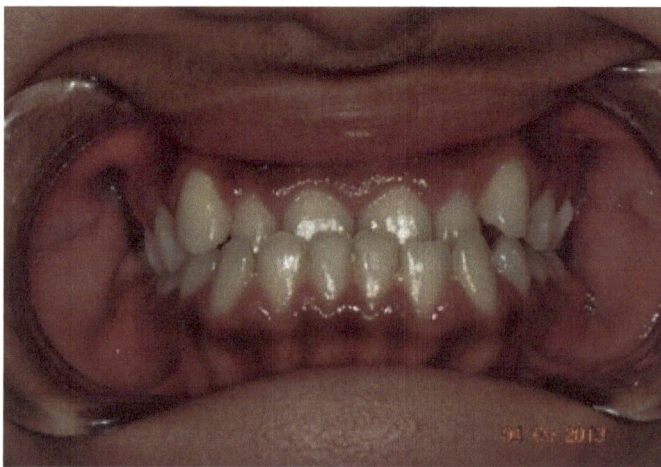

Fig. (6.15). Anterior crossbite in individual with Crouzon syndrome.

There are reports of greater maxillary retrognathism and relative mandibular prognathism in individuals with Crouzon syndrome [23]. Kreiborg and Cohen [24] stated that the differences between the two syndromes are more marked in childhood.

Dental care requires toothbrushing instructions due to the difficult dental plaque control caused by frequent tooth crowding. The plaque and gingivitis index may be high, with good indication for regular follow-up. Compliance is good, since the intellectual development is usually normal [11]; however, the dentist should consider the possibility of hypoacusia. Orthodontic management requires distraction osteogenesis or orthognathic surgery in nearly all cases, due to maxillary deficiency. Maxillary advancement may be helpful to reduce the exophthalmos by advancement of the inferior orbital rim, which is characteristically shallow. There are reports of success in the orthodontic treatment of these individuals [31].

O'Donnell [31] highlighted the need of early intervention, especially from an esthetic standpoint, aiming to increase the self-esteem of individuals. Other authors mentioned that previously these individuals were believed to have intellectual disability, which was later demonstrated not to be true, with possibility of social rather than mental disability, mentioning that due to their appearance, these individuals were often considered socially unacceptable and could not have normal social interaction [30].

PFEIFFER SYNDROME

The Pfeiffer syndrome presents autosomal dominant inheritance and is caused by mutations in the FGFR 2 gene on chromosome 10q26, and there is a subgroup of Pfeiffer syndrome with identical phenotype caused by mutation in the FGFR 1 gene at the chromosomal region 8p11.2-p11.1 [32]. The syndrome was reported by Pfeiffer [33], who described eight affected individuals in three generations. It is characterized by turribrachycephaly and may be accompanied by cloverleaf skull, coronal craniosynostosis (with or without sagittal craniosynostosis), maxillary hypoplasia and mandibular prognathism, hyperteleorbitism, shallow orbits and oblique palpebral fissures (Fig. **6.16**). There may be choanal atresia or stenosis and laryngotracheomalacia. It is differentiated from Apert syndrome by enlargement of the thumbs and big toes, with absent or partial syndactyly (Fig. **6.17**) [6, 8, 34]. Intelligence is usually normal, yet there are isolated reports of intellectual disability [6, 34].

Besides maxillary hypoplasia and mandibular prognathism, there may be high-arched palate and tooth crowding [34]. In 1993, Alvarez *et al.* [35] reported the case of a newborn of African descent with Pfeiffer syndrome type 3, who presented three natal mandibular incisors that were extracted at 4 days of age, and two natal maxillary molars that were extracted at 10 days of age. The teeth were extracted because they were immature, did not had roots and were extremely movable. The presence of several other anomalies led to death at 14 months of age due to respiratory insufficiency.

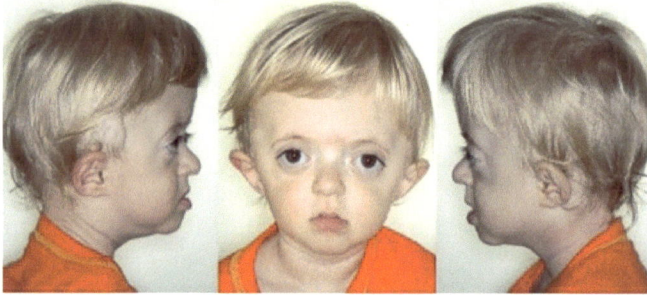

Fig. (6.16). Individual with Pfeiffer syndrome.

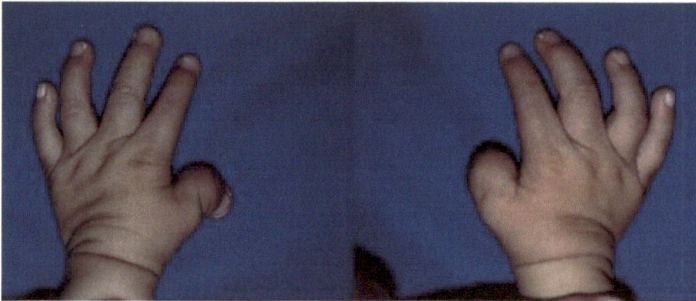

Fig. (6.17). Enlargement of the thumbs in individual with Pfeiffer syndrome.

The only study available on the oral health conditions of these individuals was conducted by Mustafa *et al.* [4] (see further information under the Apert syndrome section).

The dental treatment of individuals with Pfeiffer syndrome is essentially conventional, and they present better oral hygiene conditions compared to individuals affected by other syndromic craniosynostoses [25].

SAETHRE-CHOTZEN SYNDROME

The Saethre-Chotzen syndrome presents autosomal dominant inheritance related to chromosomal regions 10q26 and 7p21, and was described in a family by Saethre [36] and another by Chotzen [37]. It is characterized by a wide and variable array of malformations that includes craniosynostosis of the coronal, lambdoid and/or metopic sutures, plagiocephaly, brachycephaly, low hairline, facial asymmetry, eyelid ptosis, long and thin nose, nasal septum deviation, brachydactyly, partial syndactyly of soft tissue (especially affecting the second and third digits), clinodactyly of the fifth digit and skeletal anomalies. There may be reduction of ear size and hearing impairment. Other characteristics include shallow orbits, hyperteleorbitism, strabismus and lacrimal duct abnormalities. There is noticeable phenotypic variability, with possibility of association with eyelid anomalies, or similar phenotype with mutation in the FGFR 3 gene. There may also be congenital cardiac disorders. The syndrome presents high penetrance and variable expressivity. Few patients present intellectual disability [6, 38].

There may be maxillary hypoplasia, with narrow palate, and cleft palate [38]. Mustafa *et al.* [6] investigated the oral health conditions of individuals with craniosynostosis (see further information under the Apert syndrome section).

JACKSON-WEISS SYNDROME

The Jackson-Weiss syndrome presents autosomal dominant inheritance related to chromosomal regions 10q26 and 8p11.2-p11.1, being characterized by midface hypoplasia, craniosynostosis and feet anomalies with medial deviation, enlargement of the big toes and soft tissue syndactyly of the second and third toes. No significant dental abnormalities are observed [6, 39].

CARPENTER SYNDROME

Also called acrocephalopolysyndactyly, the Carpenter syndrome presents autosomal recessive inheritance. It is characterized by craniosynostosis of the sagittal and lambdoid sutures in early childhood and coronal suture in older ages, brachycephaly, midface hypoplasia, low stature, hand malformation with brachydactyly, clinodactyly and/or syndactyly and feet malformation with preaxial polysyndactyly.

The occurrence of unilateral craniosynostosis causes marked cranial asymmetry. Affected individuals present low-set ears and preauricular fistulae with possibility of conductive or sensorineural hearing loss. The eyes present epicanthal folds and there may be corneal opacity, microcornea, optical atrophy and lateral displacement of medial canthi. There may be cardiovascular, abdominal and genitourinary abnormalities, and variable delay in central nervous system development, with IQ ranging from 52 to 104. There is possibility of early puberty. It may be associated with cloverleaf skull [6, 40].

In addition to the high-arched palate and retention of deciduous teeth [40], there are reports of late tooth development with hypodontia, which the authors assigned to possible related bone disorders [40, 41]. During dental treatment, the dental professional should observe the neuropsychomotor development and consequent compliance, besides the possible hearing impairment and investigate any occasional systemic disturbances.

CLOVERLEAF SKULL

The cloverleaf skull syndrome (or Kleeblattschaedel) is very rare, with few reported cases in the literature, all of which are sporadic. The head presents a trilobular configuration, caused by hydrocephalus associated with congenital craniosynostosis of the coronal and lambdoid sutures. In more severe cases there is marked exophthalmos with corneal ulceration. There is no known genetic etiology, yet it may be observed in association with Crouzon, Pfeiffer and Carpenter syndromes [6, 42].

SHPRINTZEN-GOLDBERG SYNDROME

The Shprintzen-Goldberg syndrome, related with chromosomal region 15q21.1, was described by Shprintzen and Goldberg [43] and involves craniosynostosis associated with dolicocephaly (Fig. **6.18**), exophthalmos, telecanthus, hyperteleorbitism, proptosis, strabismus, low-set ears, multiple abdominal hernia, arachnodactyly and camptodactyly. There may be cardiovascular and genitourinary disorders. The skin is hyperelastic. There is hypotonia with possibility of delayed neuropsychomotor development. The oral findings include maxillomandibular hypoplasia, hypertrophy of the palatal mucosa, high-arched palate and malocclusion.

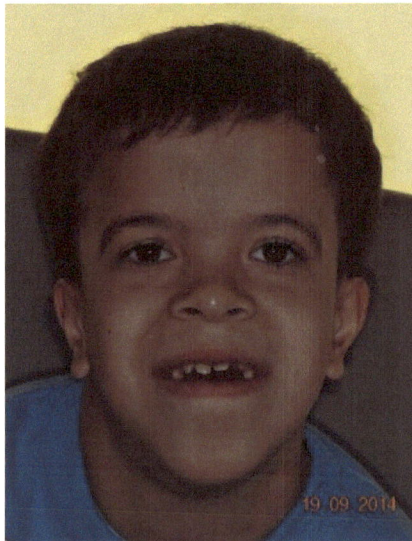

Fig. (6.18). Typical facial aspect in individual with Shprintzen-Goldberg syndrome.

ACROCRANIOFACIAL DYSOSTOSIS

This syndrome was described in two sisters, daughters of consanguineous parents by Kaplan [44], and is characterized by craniosynostosis, low stature, acrocephaly, hypoteleorbitism, proptosis, ptosis, oblique palpebral fissures, short philtrum, cleft palate, micrognathia, ear malformations, conductive or sensorineural hearing impairment, bulbous digits, pectus excavatum and partial duplication of the distal phalanx of the thumb, besides other limb anomalies [45].

CONFLICT OF INTEREST

The author (editor) declares no conflict of interest, financial or otherwise.

ACKNOWLEDGEMENTS

Declared none.

REFERENCES

[1]   Buchanan EP, Xue AS, Hollier LH Jr. Craniofacial syndromes. Plast Reconstr Surg 2014; 134(1): 128e-53e.
        [http://dx.doi.org/10.1097/PRS.0000000000000308] [PMID: 25028828]

[2]   Hamm JA, Robin NH. Newborn craniofacial malformations: orofacial clefting and craniosynostosis. Clin Perinatol 2015; 42(2): 321-336, viii.
        [http://dx.doi.org/10.1016/j.clp.2015.02.005] [PMID: 26042907]

[3]   Twigg SR, Wilkie AO. New insights into craniofacial malformations. Hum Mol Genet 2015; 24(R1): R50-9.
        [http://dx.doi.org/10.1093/hmg/ddv228] [PMID: 26085576]

[4]   Mustafa D, Lucas VS, Junod P, Evans R, Mason C, Roberts GJ. The dental health and caries-related microflora in children with craniosynostosis. Cleft Palate Craniofac J 2001; 38(6): 629-35.
        [http://dx.doi.org/10.1597/1545-1569(2001)038<0629:TDHACR>2.0.CO;2] [PMID: 11681997]

[5]   Apert ME. De l'acrocephalosyndactylie. Bull Mem Soc Med Hop Paris 1906; 23: 1310-30.

[6]   Gorlin RJ, Cohen MM Jr, Levin LS. Syndromes with craniosynostosis: general aspects and well-known syndromes. In: Gorlin RJ, Cohen MM, Hennekam RC, Eds. Syndromes of the head and neck New York. Oxford 1990; pp. 519-36.

[7]   McKusick VA. Apert syndrome. Available at: http://omim.org/entry/101200

[8]   Zanini SA. Apert, Crouzon e Pfeiffer. In: Zanini SA, Ed. Cirurgia craniofacial: malformações. Rio de Janeiro: Revinter 2000; pp. 269-76.

[9]   Letra A, de Almeida AL, Kaizer R, Esper LA, Sgarbosa S, Granjeiro JM. Intraoral features of Apert's syndrome. Oral Surg Oral Med Oral Pathol Oral Radiol Endod 2007; 103(5): e38-41.
        [http://dx.doi.org/10.1016/j.tripleo.2006.04.006] [PMID: 17466880]

[10]   Vadiati Saberi B, Shakoorpour A. Apert syndrome: report of a case with emphasis on oral manifestations. J Dent (Tehran) 2011; 8(2): 90-5.
        [PMID: 21998814]

[11]   Perosa GB. Desenvolvimento intelectual e craniossinostose. In: Zanini SA, Ed. Cirurgia craniofacial: malformações. Rio de Janeiro: Revinter 2000; pp. 145-52.

[12]   Yacubian-Fernandes A, Palhares A, Giglio A, *et al.* Apert syndrome: factors involved in the cognitive development. Arq Neuropsiquiatr 2005; 63(4): 963-8.
[http://dx.doi.org/10.1590/S0004-282X2005000600011] [PMID: 16400413]

[13]   Salinas CF. Orodental findings and genetic disorders. Birth Defects Orig Artic Ser 1982; 18(1): 79-120.
[PMID: 7115915]

[14]   Dalben GdaS, das Neves LT, Gomide MR. Oral findings in patients with Apert syndrome. J Appl Oral Sci 2006; 14(6): 465-9.
[http://dx.doi.org/10.1590/S1678-77572006000600014] [PMID: 19089249]

[15]   Kreiborg S, Cohen MM Jr. The oral manifestations of Apert syndrome. J Craniofac Genet Dev Biol 1992; 12(1): 41-8.
[PMID: 1572940]

[16]   Schudy FF. Treatment of Cruson's and Apert's syndromes. J Clin Orthod 1986; 20(2): 114-7.
[PMID: 3457800]

[17]   Kaloust S, Ishii K, Vargervik K. Dental development in Apert syndrome. Cleft Palate Craniofac J 1997; 34(2): 117-21.
[http://dx.doi.org/10.1597/1545-1569(1997)034<0117:DDIAS>2.3.CO;2] [PMID: 9138505]

[18]   Rynearson RD. Case report: orthodontic and dentofacial orthopedic considerations in Apert's syndrome. Angle Orthod 2000; 70(3): 247-52.
[PMID: 10926435]

[19]   Kreiborg S, Aduss H, Cohen MM Jr. Cephalometric study of the Apert syndrome in adolescence and adulthood. J Craniofac Genet Dev Biol 1999; 19(1): 1-11.
[PMID: 10378142]

[20]   Paravatty RP, Ahsan A, Sebastian BT, Pai KM, Dayal PK. Apert syndrome: a case report with discussion of craniofacial features. Quintessence Int 1999; 30(6): 423-6.
[PMID: 10635279]

[21]   Costaras-Volarich M, Pruzansky S. Is the mandible intrinsically different in Apert and Crouzon syndromes? Am J Orthod 1984; 85(6): 475-87.
[http://dx.doi.org/10.1016/0002-9416(84)90087-3] [PMID: 6610361]

[22]   Dalben GdaS, Costa B, Gomide MR. Oral health status of children with syndromic craniosynostosis. Oral Health Prev Dent 2006; 4(3): 173-9.
[PMID: 16961025]

[23]   Cohen MM Jr, Kreiborg S. A clinical study of the craniofacial features in Apert syndrome. Int J Oral Maxillofac Surg 1996; 25(1): 45-53.
[http://dx.doi.org/10.1016/S0901-5027(96)80011-7] [PMID: 8833300]

[24]   Kreiborg S, Cohen MM Jr. Is craniofacial morphology in Apert and Crouzon syndromes the same? Acta Odontol Scand 1998; 56(6): 339-41.
[http://dx.doi.org/10.1080/000163598428275] [PMID: 10066112]

[25]   Múfalo PS, Kaizer RdeO, Dalben GdaS, de Almeida AL. Comparison of periodontal parameters in individuals with syndromic craniosynostosis. J Appl Oral Sci 2009; 17(1): 13-20.
[http://dx.doi.org/10.1590/S1678-77572009000100004] [PMID: 19148400]

[26]   Crouzon O. Dysostose cranio-faciale hereditaire. Bull Mem Bull Mem Soc Med Hop Paris 1912; 33: 545-55.

[27]   McKusick VA. Crouzon syndrome. Available at: http://omim.org/entry/123500 1996.

[28]   Carinci F, Avantaggiato A, Curioni C. Crouzon syndrome: cephalometric analysis and evaluation of pathogenesis. Cleft Palate Craniofac J 1994; 31(3): 201-9.
[http://dx.doi.org/10.1597/1545-1569(1994)031<0201:CSCAAE>2.3.CO;2] [PMID: 8068703]

[29]   Pilger TW. The cranio-facial hereditary syndrome of Crouzon. Int J Orthod 1974; 12(3): 25-9.
        [PMID: 4607735]

[30]   Turvey TA, Long RE Jr, Hall DJ. Multidisciplinary management of Crouzon syndrome. J Am Dent
        Assoc 1979; 99(2): 205-9.
        [http://dx.doi.org/10.14219/jada.archive.1979.0253] [PMID: 379109]

[31]   O'Donnell D. Dental management problems related to self-image in Crouzon's syndrome. Aust Dent J
        1985; 30(5): 355-7.
        [http://dx.doi.org/10.1111/j.1834-7819.1985.tb02530.x] [PMID: 2937396]

[32]   McKusick VA. Shprintzen-Goldberg craniosynostosis syndrome; SGS. Available at:
        http://omim.org/entry/182212 2002b.

[33]   Pfeiffer RA. Dominant erbliche Akrocephalosyndaktylie. Z Kinderheilkd 1964; 90: 301-20.
        [http://dx.doi.org/10.1007/BF00447500] [PMID: 14316612]

[34]   McKusick VA. Pfeiffer syndrome. Available at: http://omim.org/entry/101600 1998.

[35]   Alvarez MP, Crespi PV, Shanske AL. Natal molars in Pfeiffer syndrome type 3: a case report. J Clin
        Pediatr Dent 1993; 18(1): 21-4.
        [PMID: 8110608]

[36]   Saethre M. Ein Beitrag zum Turmschaedelproblem (Pathogenese, Erblichkeit und Symptomatologie).
        Dtsch Z Nervenheilkd 1931; 119: 533-55.
        [http://dx.doi.org/10.1007/BF01673869]

[37]   Chotzen F. Eine eigenartige familiaere Entwicklungsstoerung (Akrocephalosyndaktylie, Dysostosis
        craniofacialis und Hypertelorismus). Mschr Kinderheilk 1932; 55: 97-122.

[38]   McKusick VA. Saethre-Chotzen syndrome; SCS. Available at: http://omim.org/entry/101400 2002a.

[39]   McKusick VA. Jackson-Weiss syndrome; JWS. Available at: http://omim.org/entry/123150 2003.

[40]   McKusick VA. Carpenter syndrome; CRPT1. Available at: http://omim.org/entry/201000 1986a.

[41]   Blankenstein R, Brook AH, Smith RN, Patrick D, Russell JM. Oral findings in Carpenter syndrome.
        Int J Paediatr Dent 2001; 11(5): 352-60.
        [http://dx.doi.org/10.1046/j.0960-7439.2001.00295.x] [PMID: 11572266]

[42]   McKusick VA. Kleeblattschaedel. Available at: http://omim.org/entry/148800 1986b.

[43]   Shprintzen RJ, Goldberg RB. A recurrent pattern syndrome of craniosynostosis associated with
        arachnodactyly and abdominal hernias. J Craniofac Genet Dev Biol 1982; 2(1): 65-74.
        [PMID: 6182156]

[44]   Kaplan P, Plauchu H, Fitch N, Jéquier S. A new acro-cranio-facial dysostosis syndrome in sisters. Am
        J Med Genet 1988; 29(1): 95-106.
        [http://dx.doi.org/10.1002/ajmg.1320290112] [PMID: 3344780]

[45]   McKusick VA. Acrocraniofacial dysostosis. Available at: http://omim.org/entry/201050 1988.

CHAPTER 7

Pharyngeal Arch Disorders

Marcia Ribeiro Gomide*

Hospital for Rehabilitation of Craniofacial Anomalies, University of São Paulo, Brazil

Abstract: The pharyngeal arches develop in the human embryo around five weeks of pregnancy. Disorders in the development of the first and second pharyngeal arches may lead to significant malformations of the face and ears. Syndromes involving the pharyngeal arches often involve tooth abnormalities, requiring regular dental follow-up with specialized management by a multidisciplinary team.

Keywords: Acrofacial dysostosis, Dental care, Goldenhar syndrome, Mandibulofacial dysostosis, Nager type, Tooth abnormalities.

The pharyngeal arches appear in mankind between the 4th to 5th week of intrauterine life, consisting of a series of structures that participate in head and neck development. These structures form laterally to the pharyngeal gut and comprise a center of mesenchymal tissue, which involves muscular, nervous and vascular components, covered by ectoderm and internally by endoderm.[2] When some of these structures are altered, especially the 1st and 2nd pharyngeal arches, which are involved in formation of the face and ears, there may be interference with their constitution resulting in anomalies and malformations in these regions.

TREACHER COLLINS SYNDROME

The Treacher Collins syndrome is one of the disorders affecting the 1st and 2nd pharyngeal arches, also called mandibulofacial dysostosis or Franceschetti syndrome. It is an autosomal dominant disorder of craniofacial development related to chromosomal region 5q32-q33.1 [1 - 4].

The prevalence of the syndrome is 1/50,000 livebirths and it is estimated that 40% of cases present familial history, with the remaining 60% being considered new mutations [4]. It presents clinical and genetic heterogeneity.

* **Corresponding author Marcia Ribeiro Gomide:** Hospital for Rehabilitation of Craniofacial Anomalies, University of São Paulo, Bauru, Brazil; Tel/Fax: +55 14 3235-8000; E-mails: marcinha@usp.br; magomide@yahoo.com.br; marcinhargomide@gmail.com

The facial aspect is peculiar (Figs. **7.1** and **7.3**) and may be detected prenatally by ultrasound, which allows observation of the face and also of the ear malformation (Figs. **7.2** and **7.4**) of variable aspect, with possible conductive hearing loss. There may be oblique palpebral clefts, upper eyelid coloboma, partial absence of lower eyelashes, and hypoplasia of the mandible and zygomatic complex. Involvement of the zygomatic region may be understood as a combination of Tessier clefts # 6, 7 and 8 [4 - 6]. The alterations are usually bilateral and symmetrical.

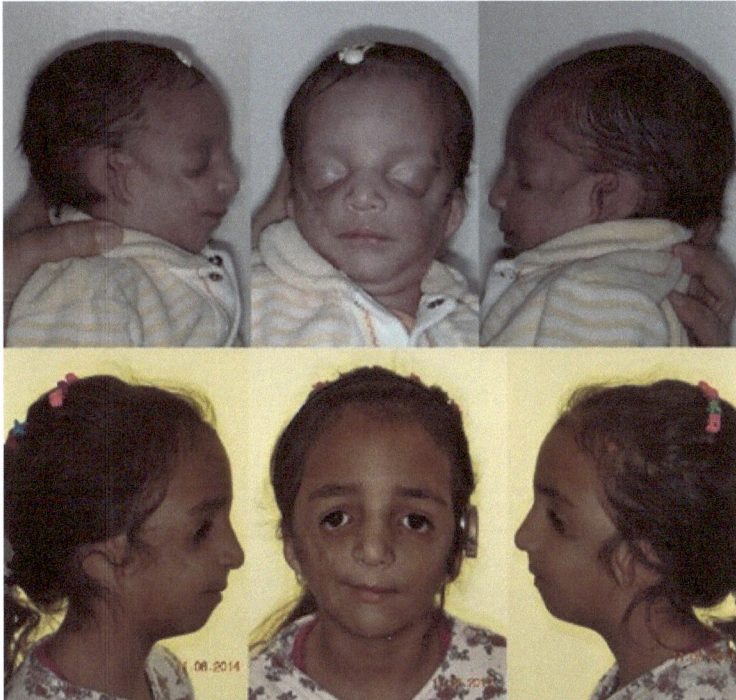

Fig. (7.1). Frontal and lateral facial aspects of individual with Treacher Collins syndrome, at two different ages. Notice maintenance of the syndromic features over time.

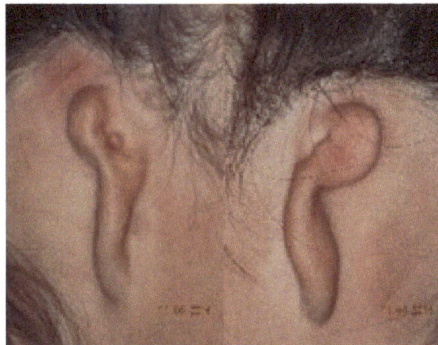

Fig. (7.2). Ear malformation in the same individual presented in Fig. (**7.1**).

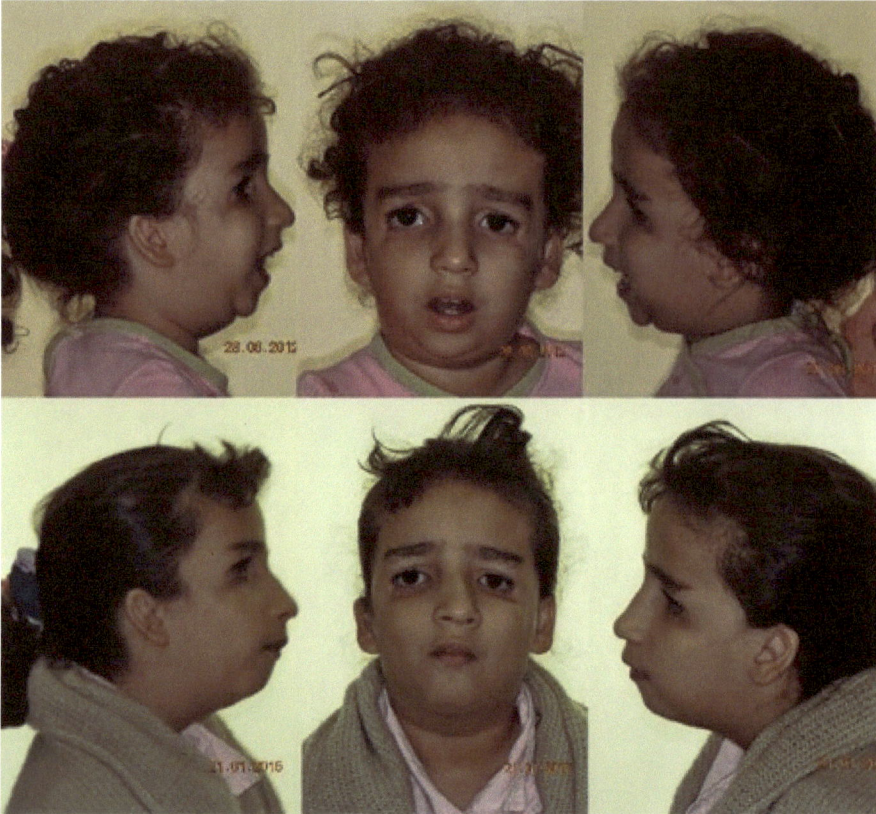

Fig. (7.3). Frontal and lateral facial aspects of individual with Treacher Collins syndrome, at two different ages. Notice maintenance of the syndromic features over time.

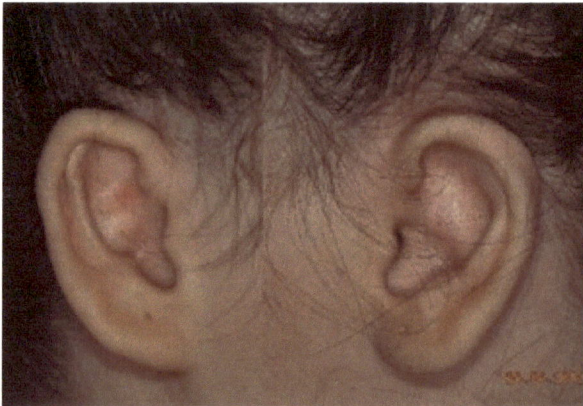

Fig. (7.4). Ear malformation in the same individual presented in Fig. **(7.3)**.

With regard to the orodental aspects, there may be hypodontia, macrostomia and cleft palate or cleft lip and palate [4 - 6]. There may be anterior open bite, maxillary biprotrusion and limited retropharyngeal space that may impair the teeth and occlusion. Individuals also present micrognathia (Fig. **7.5**) [7 - 9], dysplasia of the temporomandibular joint, limited mouth opening, midline deviation (Figs. **7.6** and **7.7**), lack of occlusion on the right side, deep bite, Class II [19] or III [7] malocclusion, mandibular rotation, mandibular retrognathism, clockwise mandibular rotation, open gonial angle, anterior open bite, maxillary prognathism or retrognathism in relation to the cranial base, and mandibular retrognathism with relative maxillary prognathism [10]. Studies evidence few alterations in skeletal morphology and growth, with marked changes in maxillary and mandibular positioning and tendency of maintenance of the syndromic facial features over time (Figs. **7.1** and **7.3**) [9]. There are reports of impacted supernumerary teeth at the maxillary anterior region, hypoplasia and malpositioning of maxillary central incisors [7]. The dental treatment of individuals with Treacher Collins syndrome may be complicated due to child's anxiety, secondary to the hearing impairment and also to micrognathia, which predisposes to breathing difficulty. For these reasons, some individuals may require dental treatment under general anesthesia, which may also be complicated yet safer than intervention under local anesthesia or sedation. These difficulties highlight the need to emphasize the importance of oral hygiene for the parents of these individuals [11]. It is always important to know the behavioral and psychological limitations of the child before intervention, adapting the treatment to his or her possibilities and enhancing the compliance.

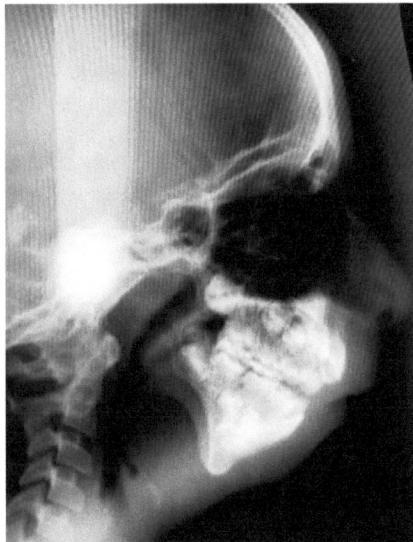

Fig. (7.5). Lateral cephalogram of individual with Treacher Collins syndrome. Notice the marked mandibular rotation and decreased airway space.

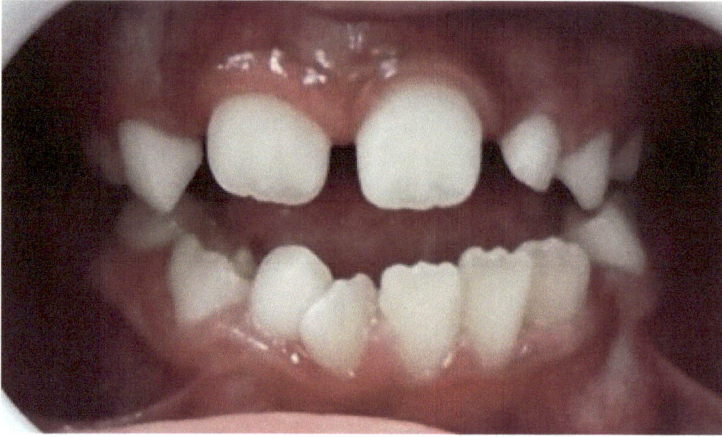

Fig. (7.6). Anterior open bite and midline deviation in individual with Treacher Collins syndrome.

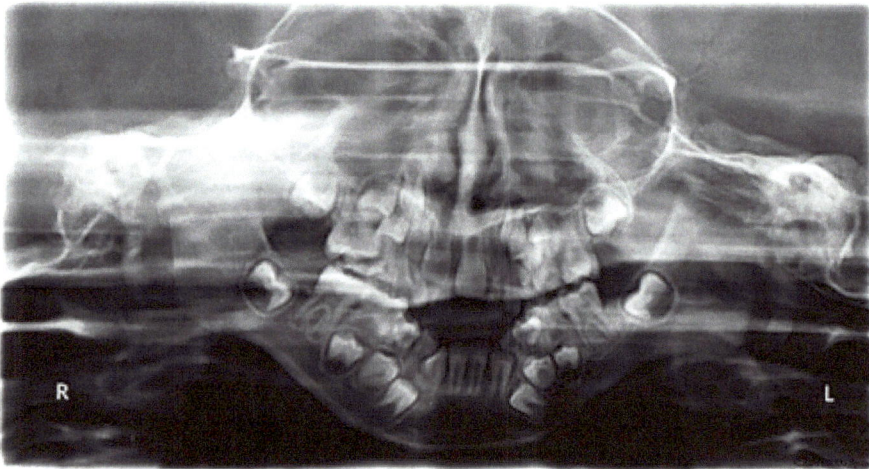

Fig. (7.7). Panoramic radiograph of the same individual with Treacher Collins syndrome presented in Fig. (**7.6**). Notice the skeletal involvement in the anterior open bite.

NAGER SYNDROME

The Nager syndrome, also called acrofacial dysostosis, is caused by a heterozygous mutation in the SF3B4 gene (OMIM 01/12/2015). Both autosomal dominant and recessive inheritances have been reported, with alteration in chromosome 9q32 and deletion of 1q12q21. The prevalence is unknown, since only 100 cases of the syndrome have been published so far [12, 13]. It was recognized as a specific disorder by Nager and Reynier [14], yet it had been probably described by Slingenberg [15]. It is differentiated from mandibulofacial dysostosis (Treacher Collins syndrome) by the presence of limb malformations. It may be detected prenatally. The face is similar to the Treacher Collins syndrome, with microcephaly, micrognathia, zygomatic hypoplasia, oblique palpebral fissures, lower eyelid coloboma and reduced number of lower eyelashes, as well as low stature and thumb hypoplasia or aplasia. Some individuals may present thumb duplication or triphalangia. The thumb anomalies are usually asymmetric. Individuals may also present syndactyly or clinodactyly. Some individuals present external ear anomalies and cleft palate, even though they are more common in Treacher Collins syndrome. There may be conductive hearing loss with low-set ears and atresia of the external auditory canal. Laryngeal and epiglottal hypoplasia have been reported. There may also be cardiovascular, respiratory, abdominal, genitourinary and neurological abnormalities (with normal intelligence and delayed speech development) and diverse skeletal anomalies [5, 16].

Concerning the oral aspects, individuals with Nager syndrome usually present more severe micrognathia compared to Treacher Collins syndrome. This characteristic, combined to the alteration of upper limbs, may complicate the oral hygiene control. Macrostomia and trismus may be observed. Tooth crowding are common, as well as deficient maxillomandibular relationship [12, 13]. Dental treatment under general anesthesia may be necessary if the access to posterior teeth is complicated by the limited mouth opening. Cleft palate may be present and its consequences should be followed and treated accordingly. Dental professionals should investigate the presence of hearing impairment, which may affect the patient compliance, and possible systemic disorders. Therefore, professionals should know the individual both physically and psychologically to offer the best treatment.

MILLER SYNDROME

Also called postaxial acrofacial dysostosis, Wildervanck-Smith or Genee-Wiedemann syndrome, the Miller syndrome presents autosomal recessive inheritance. It was described by Miller [17], even though several authors reported individuals with the syndrome previously. The syndrome is caused by a mutation in the DHODH gene in chromosome 16q22 [18]. The facial aspect is similar to the Treacher Collins syndrome, being differentiated by the presence of postaxial limb anomalies, mainly postaxial agenesis of one finger or toe. The thumbs are abnormal in 50% if cases. There is maxillary hypoplasia with oblique palpebral fissures. The eyelids may present coloboma and there is usually ectropium of the lower eyelids. Individuals may also present abdominal, genitourinary and skeletal anomalies [5, 17 - 21].

Concerning the orodental aspects, in addition to the severe micrognathia and cleft lip and/or palate, the individuals may present consequences of these alterations, such as tooth crowding. Peg-shaped teeth were also reported [5, 20]. Oral hygiene control may be impaired due to physical limitations.

OCULOAURICULOVERTEBRAL SPECTRUM

The oculoauriculovertebral spectrum, also called hemifacial microsomia, oculoauriculovertebral dysplasia or Goldenhar syndrome, is an autosomal dominant disorder associated with chromosomal region 14q32 [22]. It is relatively frequent, affecting approximately 1 in every 5,600 births. The male to female ratio is at least 3:2, with predilection for the right side also in a ratio of 3:2. This is a primary developmental disorder affecting structures derived from the first and second pharyngeal arches during embryogenesis [23]. The phenotype is widely variable, with craniofacial anomalies, cardiovascular, respiratory, genitourinary, vertebral (anomalies and hypoplasia) and central nervous system abnormalities, with possible intellectual impairment, hydrocephalus and occipital hydrocephaly. The disorder is often unilateral (70 to 90%). Most cases are sporadic, yet there are reports of familial recurrence [5, 22]. There are reports of association with maternal diabetes and utilization of thalidomide, primidone and retinoic acid [24].

The craniofacial characteristics include marked facial asymmetry (Figs. **7.8** and **7.10**) due to underlying skeletal anomalies, which may not be visible in childhood yet may become apparent during growth, usually appearing at four years of age. The soft tissues may mask the skeletal asymmetry; conversely, a deficient soft tissue volume may also cause facial asymmetry over adequate bone structures. The maxillary and temporal bones on the more severely affected side present reduced size and flattening. The asymmetry may also be caused by aplasia or hypoplasia of the mandibular ramus and condyle (Figs. **7.8** and **7.9**). The facial musculature is hypoplastic. The eye abnormalities may include upper eyelid coloboma (Fig. **7.8**), blepharophimosis, microphthalmia, anophthalmia and strabismus. The phenotype is clinically heterogeneous and is typically characterized by abnormal ear development with possibility of mild ear deformity, preauricular tags (Figs. **7.8** and **7.10**), preauricular sinuses, atresia of the external auditory canal, microtia (Figs. **7.8** and **7.10**), anotia and conductive hearing loss [25]. The neck may present branchial cleft [5, 22].

Concerning orodental aspects, there may be macrostomia, cleft lip and/or palate, besides reports of bifid tongue, maxillary and mandibular hypoplasia, malocclusion, tooth-size discrepancy, hypodontia of second premolars and third molars, supernumerary teeth, enamel defects and delayed tooth development. Proper treatment depends on observation of the diverse anomalies and physical and behavioral limitations of each individual, with special emphasis to positioning in the dental chair due to the increased risk of atlantoaxial instability, which may be lethal if not properly managed [26].

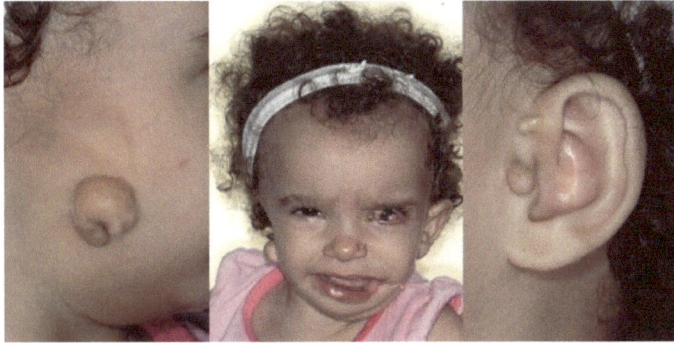

Fig. (7.8). Individual with oculoauriculovertebral spectrum. Notice the asymmetric eye and ear abnormalities, with microtia on the right side and preauricular tags on the left side; and macrostomia on the left side.

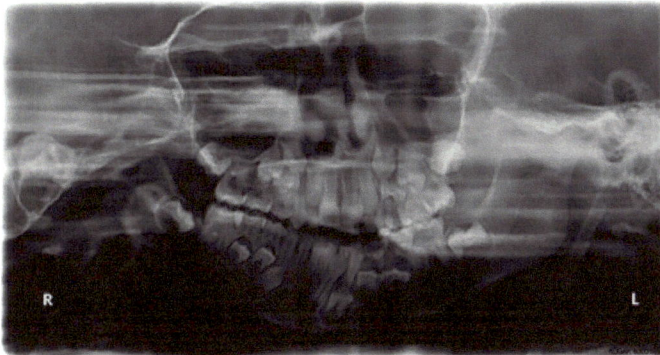

Fig. (7.9). Panoramic radiograph of the same individual with oculoauriculovertebral spectrum. Notice the marked mandibular asymmetry, which is more promptly visible radiographically than clinically.

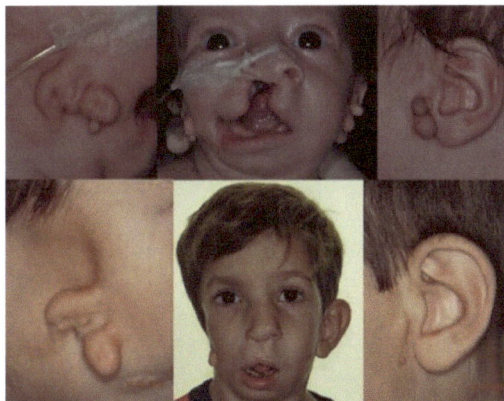

Fig. (7.10). Individual with oculoauriculovertebral spectrum. Alike Fig. (**7.8**), this presents asymmetrical ear abnormalities, with microtia on the right side and preauricular tags on the left side, without eye anomalies and with complete right cleft lip and palate, evidencing the phenotypic variability. The photographs present two different ages; the second row exhibits the aspect after surgical correction of cleft lip and palate and preauricular tags. Notice worsening of facial asymmetry during growth.

CONFLICT OF INTEREST

The author (editor) declares no conflict of interest, financial or otherwise.

ACKNOWLEDGEMENTS

Declared none.

REFERENCES

[1]   da Silva Dalben G, Teixeira das Neves L, Ribeiro Gomide M. Oral health status of children with treacher Collins syndrome. Spec Care Dentist 2006; 26(2): 71-5.
        [http://dx.doi.org/10.1111/j.1754-4505.2006.tb01513.x] [PMID: 16681242]

[2]   Mohan RPS, Verma S, Agarwal N, Singh U. Treacher Collins syndrome: a case report. BMJ Case Rep 2013.
        [http://dx.doi.org/10.1136/bcr-2013-009341]

[3]   Ranadheer E, Nagaraju K, Suresh P, Updesh M. Eight year follow-up dental treatment in a patient with Treacher Collins syndrome. J Indian Soc Pedod Prev Dent 2012; 30(3): 254-7.
        [http://dx.doi.org/10.4103/0970-4388.105020] [PMID: 23263431]

[4]   Zanini SA. Disostoses mandibulofaciais ou síndrome de Treacher Collins. In: Zanini SA, Ed. Cirurgia craniofacial: malformações. Rio de Janeiro: Revinter 2000; pp. 223-7.

[5]   Gorlin RJ, Cohen MM Junior, Levin LS. Branchial arch and oro-acral disorders. In: Gorlin RJ, Cohen MM, Hennekam RC, Eds. Syndromes of the head and neck New York. Oxford 1990; pp. 641-54.

[6]   McKusick VA. Treacher Collins-Franceschetti syndrome 1; TCS1. Available at: http://omim.org/entry/154500 2002c.

[7]   Anil S, Beena VT, Ankathil R, Remani P, Vijayakumar T. Mandibulofacial dysostosis. Case report. Aust Dent J 1995; 40(1): 39-42.
        [http://dx.doi.org/10.1111/j.1834-7819.1995.tb05612.x] [PMID: 7710415]

[8]   Opitz C. Kieferorthopädische Behandlung bei dem Formenkreis der Dysostosis mandibulo-facialis. Stomatol DDR 1978; 28(6): 405-9.
        [PMID: 276961]

[9]   Rune B, Sarnäs KV, Aberg M. Mandibulofacial dysostosis--variability in facial morphology and growth: a long-term profile roentgenographic and roentgen stereometric analysis of three patients. Cleft Palate Craniofac J 1999; 36(2): 110-22.
        [http://dx.doi.org/10.1597/1545-1569(1999)036<0110:MDVIFM>2.3.CO;2] [PMID: 10213056]

[10]   Goldberg JS, Enlow DH, Whitaker LA, Zins JE, Kurihara S. Some anatomical characteristics in several craniofacial syndromes. J Oral Surg 1981; 39(7): 489-98.
        [PMID: 6940956]

[11]   Shapira J, Gleicher H, Moskovitz M, Peretz B. Respiratory arrest in Treacher-Collins syndrome: implications for dental management: case report. Pediatr Dent 1996; 18(3): 242-4.
        [PMID: 8784917]

[12]   Abdollahi Fakhim S, Shahidi N, Mousaviagdas M. A case report: nager acrofacial dysostosis. Iran J Otorhinolaryngol 2012; 24(66): 45-50.
        [PMID: 24303385]

[13]   Bozatlıoğlu R, Münevveroğlu AP. Dental management of a patient with Nager acrofacial dysostosis. Case Rep Dent 2015; 2015: 984732.
        [http://dx.doi.org/10.1155/2015/984732]

[14]   Nager FR, Reynier JP. Das Gehörorgan bei den angeborenen Kopfmissbildungen. Pract Otorhinolaryngol (Basel) 1948; 2 (Suppl. 2): 1-128.

[15]   Missbildungen von Extremitäten SB. Virchows Arch Pathol Anat Physiol Klin Med 1908; 193: 1-91. [http://dx.doi.org/10.1007/BF01991532]

[16]   McKusick VA. Acrofacial dysostosis 1, Nager Type; AFD1. Available at: http://omim.org/ entry/154400 2003.

[17]   Miller M, Fineman R, Smith DW. Postaxial acrofacial dysostosis syndrome. J Pediatr 1979; 95(6): 970-5. [http://dx.doi.org/10.1016/S0022-3476(79)80285-1] [PMID: 501501]

[18]   Fang J, Uchiumi T, Yagi M, *et al.* Dihydro-orotate dehydrogenase is physically associated with the respiratory complex and its loss leads to mitochondrial dysfunction. Biosci Rep 2013; 33(2): e00021. [http://dx.doi.org/10.1042/BSR20120097] [PMID: 23216091]

[19]   Genée E. Une forme extensive de dysostose mandibulo-faciale. J Genet Hum 1969; 17(1): 45-52. [PMID: 5808539]

[20]   McKusick VA. Postaxial acrofacial dysostosis; POADS. Available at: http://omim.org/entry/263750 2002b.

[21]   Wiedemann HR. Mibbbildungs-Retardierungs-Syndrom mit Fehlen des 5. Strahls an Händen und Fübben, Gaumenspalte, dysplastischen Ohren und Augenlidern und radioulnarer Synostose. Klin Padiatr 1973; 185(3): 181-6. [PMID: 4795571]

[22]   McKusick VA. Hemifacial microsomia; HFM. Available at: http://omim.org/entry/263750 2002a.

[23]   Beleza-Meireles A, Clayton-Smith J, Saraiva JM, Tassabehji M. Oculo-auriculo-vertebral spectrum: a review of the literature and genetic update. J Med Genet 2014; 51(10): 635-45. [http://dx.doi.org/10.1136/jmedgenet-2014-102476] [PMID: 25118188]

[24]   Collares MV. Displasias mandibulofaciais. In: Zanini SA, Ed. Cirurgia craniofacial: malformações. Rio de Janeiro: Revinter 2000; pp. 229-40.

[25]   Bogusiak K, Arkuszewski P, Skorek-Stachnik K, Kozakiewicz M. Treatment strategy in Goldenhar syndrome. J Craniofac Surg 2014; 25(1): 177-83. [http://dx.doi.org/10.1097/SCS.0000000000000387] [PMID: 24406574]

[26]   McKay SD, Al-Omari A, Tomlinson LA, Dormans JP. Review of cervical spine anomalies in genetic syndromes. Spine 2012; 37(5): E269-77. [http://dx.doi.org/10.1097/BRS.0b013e31823b3ded] [PMID: 22045003]

CHAPTER 8

Syndromes with Characteristic Facies

Marcia Ribeiro Gomide[*], Gisele da Silva Dalben[*] and Lucimara Teixeira das Neves[*]

Bauru School of Dentistry and Hospital for Rehabilitation of Craniofacial Anomalies, University of São Paulo, Brazil

Abstract: A wide array of syndromes reported in the literature have significant impact on the craniofacial complex, with great influence on the facial aspect, which is usually typical of each syndrome. For this reason, this chapter refers to these disorders as "syndromes with unusual facies", as described in the classical book of Gorlin *et al.,*. Affecting the craniofacial complex, these syndromes also often have significant implications for dental treatment and affected individuals may have peculiar dental needs.

Keywords: Autosomal dominant, Autosomal recessive, Craniofrontonasal dysplasia, De Lange syndrome, Dental care, Frontonasal dysplasia, Fronto-faci--nasal dysplasia, Kabuki syndrome, Mobius syndrome, Opitz GBBB syndrome, Robinow syndrome, Tooth abnormalities, X-linked.

FRONTONASAL DYSPLASIA

Frontonasal dysplasia is a craniofacial midline defect, involving combinations of the following characteristics: hyperteleorbitism; broad nasal base; unilateral or bilateral alar cleft; absent nasal tip; and widow's peak [1, 2] (Figs. **8.1** and **8.2**). The associated defects may include median cleft of the nose and/or upper lip (Fig. **8.3**) and rarely of the palate. The individuals may present low-set ears, ear tags, absent tragus and conductive hearing loss. In addition to hyperteleorbitism, there may be lateral displacement of the internal canthi with secondary telecanthus, microphthalmia, epicanthal folds, ptosis, coloboma and cataract. The nose may be bifid to variable extents (Fig. **8.3**).

[*] **Corresponding author Marcia Ribeiro Gomide:** Hospital for Rehabilitation of Craniofacial Anomalies, University of São Paulo, Bauru, Brazil; Tel/Fax: +55 14 3235-8000; E-mail: marcinha@usp.br
[*] **Gisele da Silva Dalben:** Hospital for Rehabilitation of Craniofacial Anomalies, University of São Paulo, Bauru, Brazil; Tel/Fax: +55 14 3235-8000; E-mail: gsdalben@usp.br
[*] **Lucimara Teixeira das Neves:** Bauru School of Dentistry and Hospital for Rehabilitation of Craniofacial Anomalies, University of São Paulo, Bauru, Brazil; Tel/Fax: +55 14 3235-8000; E-mail: lucimaraneves@fob.usp.br

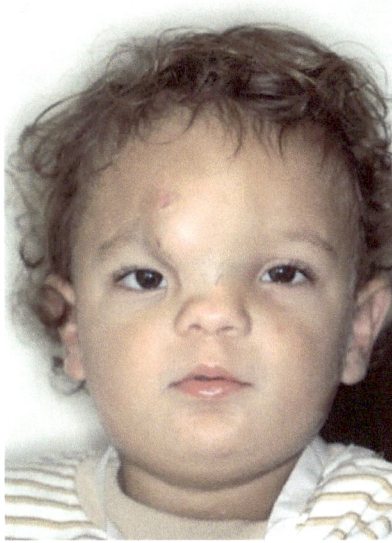

Fig. (8.1). Individual with frontonasal dysplasia exhibiting hyperteleorbitism, broad nasal base and encephalocele.

There may also be tetralogy of Fallot, frontal cutaneous lipoma, hypoplasia or aplasia of the pectoralis muscle, maxillary hypoplasia and hypoplastic frontal sinuses.

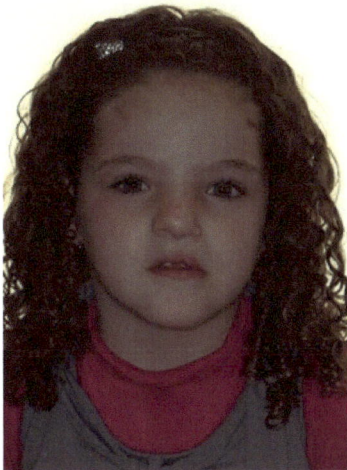

Fig. (8.2). Individual with frontonasal dysplasia exhibiting hyperteleorbitism. Notice the mild phenotype as compared to the individual presented in Fig. (**8.1**).

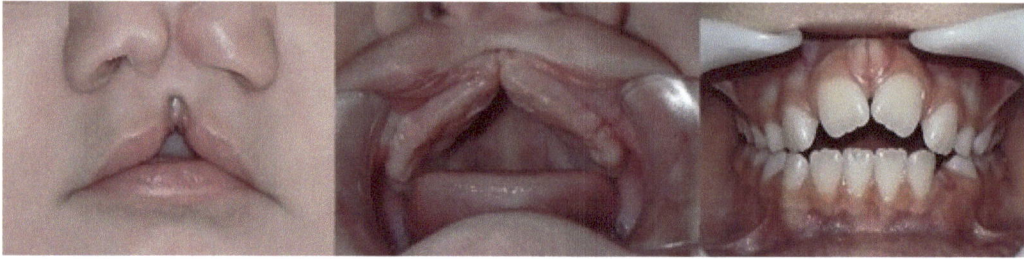

Fig. (8.3). Bifid nose and midline alveolar cleft in individual with frontonasal dysplasia. On the right side, notice the V-shaped anterior open bite at a later age.

There may be occult anterior bifid cranium with possibility of intellectual disability, lipoma or agenesis of the corpus callosum and basal anterior encephalocele (Fig. **8.1**). The intellectual development may vary from normal to severe intellectual disability, yet most individuals present normal intelligence. Intellectual disability seems to be related with extra-encephalic disorders or severe hyperteleorbitism [3].

Even though the etiology of frontonasal dysplasia is unknown, there are reports of association with teratogenic drugs, autosomal dominant inheritance, multifactorial transmission and polygenic inheritance. Studies in animal models suggested that genetic inhibitors were associated with the syndrome, and genes participating in human embryogenesis might be affected in the craniofacial midline syndrome.

It is necessary to analyze the individual with frontonasal dysplasia from a behavioral standpoint; as previously mentioned, the intelligence may be normal or abnormal. Preparation of the individual to achieve compliance with dental treatment is important and necessary. However, most individuals present normal behavior, allowing conventional dental treatment. Little information is available in the literature about the oral characteristics specific of individuals with frontonasal dysplasia. Similar to the wide diversity of craniofacial phenotypes in this syndrome, the same is observed for orodental findings (Fig. **8.4**); apparently, the dental disorders seem to be related with clefts accompanying the syndrome, causing enamel hypoplasia, double teeth, ectopic eruption of permanent first molars, hypodontia of premolars and lateral incisors [1]. Anterior open bite and interincisal diastema are observed in case of anterior clefts.

Orthodontic and orthognathic treatment are performed as necessary based on the treatment planning, according to the clinical and radiographic diagnosis. These procedures may be complex when the alveolar median cleft is wide, evidencing the importance of proper diagnosis and treatment planning.

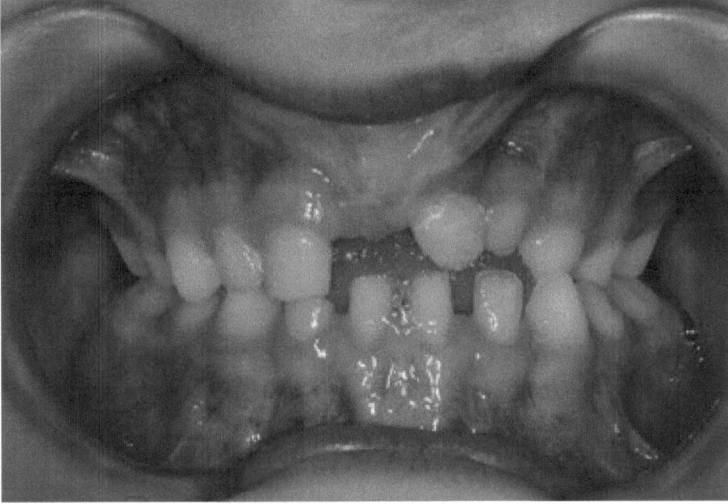

Fig. (8.4). Interincisal diastema in the same individual with frontonasal dysplasia presented in Fig. (**8.2**). Notice this remarkable orodental finding, despite the mild facial manifestations.

CRANIOFRONTONASAL DYSPLASIA

Craniofrontonasal dysplasia, also called craniofrontal syndrome or craniofrontal dysostosis, may be caused by a mutation in the EFNB1 gene on chromosome Xq12 [4]. It is a X-linked developmental disorder that paradoxically presents greater severity in heterozygous females than in homozygous males. The females present frontonasal dysplasia, craniofacial asymmetry, craniosynostosis, bifid nasal tip, grooved nails and other digit anomalies as syndactyly and clinodactyly of the fifth digit, thick and wiry hair, and abnormalities of thoracic skeleton. There are frequent reports of strabismus and facial asymmetry, telecanthus, exotropia and nystagmus, with occasional cases of unilateral or bilateral cleft lip and palate. Other findings include narrow shoulders. Males typically present hyperteleorbitism [5, 6], brachydactyly, syndactyly and broad halluces [3]. There are also reports of low stature; the diagnosis of males with this disorder requires radiographic observation of increased bone distance between the orbits. The systemic abnormalities include umbilical hernia, hypospadia, short limbs, joint hypermobility, hypotonia and hypoplasia of the corpus callosum [3]. The intelligence is usually normal, with possibility of intellectual disability in females [3].

Dental professionals should be attentive to the individual's behavior to enhance the compliance. Dental treatment may be performed as usual, and there are no reports in the literature about specific dental features in this syndrome. There may be orodental manifestations related to the cleft, when present, and in such cases the dental and orthodontic/orthognathic treatment are related to this aspect, including hypoplastic, supernumerary and malpositioned teeth close to the cleft affecting the alveolar ridge.

FRONTOFACIONASAL DYSPLASIA

The frontofacionasal dysplasia or frontofacionasal dysostosis is a rare genetic disorder present at birth, described by Gollop in 1981 [7], primarily characterized by brachycephaly, occult bifid cranium, blepharophimosis, palpebral ptosis, lagophthalmos of the lower eyelid (inability to completely close the eyes), telecanthus, S-shaped palpebral fissures, hypoplastic midface and cleft lip and palate [8]. There may also be hypoplasia of the frontal bone, absent eyelashes, cataract, microphthalmia, microcornea and nasal hypoplasia. There may be eye abnormalities as coloboma of the upper eyelid or of the iris. The frontofacionasal dysplasia seems to present autosomal recessive inheritance [3], with reported prevalence of 1:100,000 to 1:120,000.

The frontofacionasal dysplasia usually does not affect the neurological development, and from the standpoint of dental care the individuals may be treated conventionally. If the individual presents cleft lip and palate affecting the alveolar ridge, there may be dental disorders as hypodontia, supernumerary teeth, enamel hypoplasia, and others. They may also require orthodontic/orthognathic procedures according to their craniofacial anatomical alterations. Preventive dental care is always recommended.

ACROFRONTOFACIONASAL DYSPLASIA

The acrofrontofacionasal dysplasia was described by Richieri-Costa *et al.,* in 1985 [9] in two siblings whose parents were first-degree cousins. The individuals presented microbrachycephaly, broad forehead, bilateral cleft lip and palate, intellectual disability, hyperteleorbitism, S-shaped palpebral fissures, ptosis, long eyelashes and eyebrows, macrostomia, polysyndactyly of the hands, hypoplasia of distal phalanges, short legs and hypospadia [3]. The occurrence in children of consanguineous parents suggests autosomal recessive inheritance. The chromosomes were normal. Naguib [10] and Chaabouni *et al.,* [11] also described similar cases in babies born to consanguineous parents.

The degree of intellectual disability should be considered in dental planning, prevention and treatment. The presence of cleft lip and palate causes inherent characteristics as hypodontia, hypoplastic, supernumerary and malpositioned teeth. The possibility of dental treatment depends on the extent of compliance.

OPITZ SYNDROME

The Optiz syndrome, also called G/BBB syndrome representing the initials of surnames of families reported with this syndrome, is a genetic disorder that causes several abnormalities along the midline, including hyperteleorbitism (Fig. **8.5**), telecanthus, hypospadia, cleft lip and palate (Fig. **8.5**) and laryngotracheopharyngeal abnormalities. From a neurological standpoint, there may be agenesis of the corpus callosum and developmental delay. The possible systemic disorders include cardiac defects, respiratory problems, imperforate anus, cryptorchidism and gastroesophageal reflux [12].

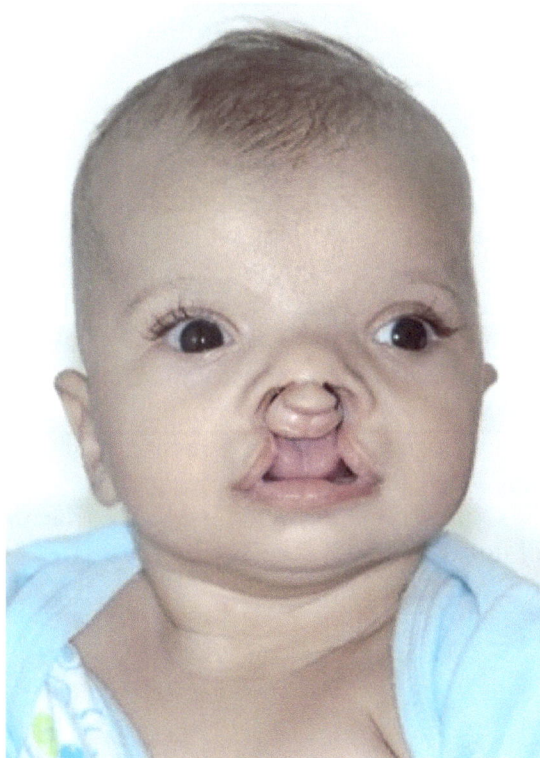

Fig. (8.5). Marked hyperteleorbitism and complete bilateral cleft lip and palate in individual with G/BBB syndrome.

Two different types of Optiz syndrome have been described on the basis of the inheritance pattern, though presenting the same signs and symptoms. One type is an X-linked syndrome caused by mutation in the MID1 gene, while the autosomal dominant syndrome type is caused by a mutation in the SPECC1L gene. Though underestimated, the estimated prevalence of the X-linked Opitz syndrome is 1:10,000 to 50,000 and the prevalence of the autosomal dominant type is unknown. However, the prevalence of the 22q11.2 deletion syndrome, to which it is related, is around 1:4,000.

Dental professionals should be attentive to the neurological and behavioral conditions of the individual during outpatient dental care, reminding that preparation and information of the individual for treatment enhances the compliance for the long rehabilitation process. Preventive procedures promote the establishment of good oral hygiene habits and may also improve the compliance. Dental treatment may be performed conventionally and depends on the type of cleft. Orodental manifestations may include micrognathia, with reports of reduced mandibular length [3, 13, 14], double teeth, supernumerary teeth [3, 14], and malocclusion. There may also be bifid uvula, bifid tongue and ankyloglossia [3, 14].

The study conducted by Dalben *et al.,* [14] revealed tooth abnormalities in 95.23% of a sample of individuals with Opitz syndrome. In this study, the most interesting findings were the presence of ankyloglossia and a supernumerary tooth in the mandibular anterior region, both of which affected 52% of individuals analyzed. These findings evidence the midline involvement inherent to the Opitz syndrome. During that study, several mothers of individuals reported also having ankyloglossia (Fig. **8.6**), highlighting the X-linked inheritance of the syndrome, in which the mothers may present milder manifestations than their male offspring. Concerning the supernumerary teeth in the mandibular anterior region, they presented as five mandibular incisors all of which exhibited normal shape and alignment (Figs. **8.7** and **8.8**), leading the present authors to conclude that the supernumerary tooth was probably the tooth located in the midline, coincident with the developmental field affected by the syndrome.

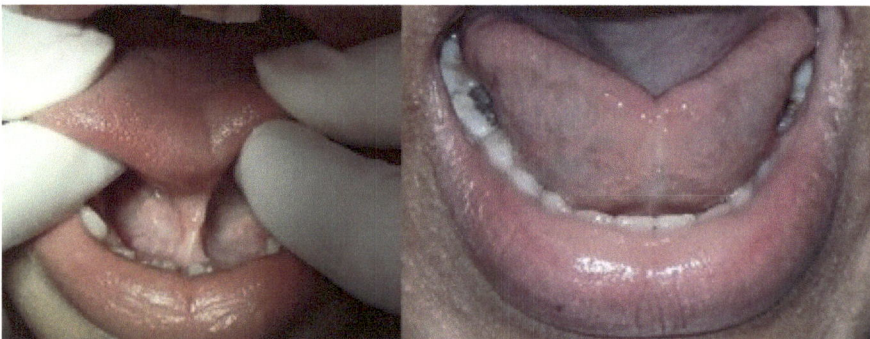

Fig. (8.6). Short lingual frenum in the same individual with G/BBB syndrome presented in Fig. (**8.5**) (left side) and in his mother (right side).

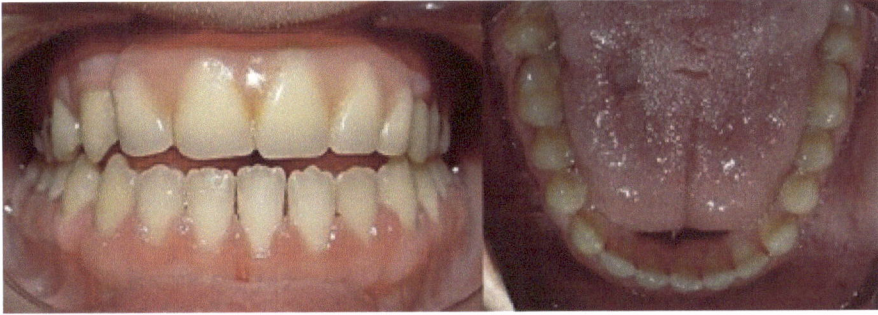

Fig. (8.7). Supernumerary mandibular incisor in individual with G/BBB syndrome. Notice the normal shape and size and good tooth alignment, despite the presence of five mandibular incisors. The supernumerary tooth is probably the tooth located in the midline.

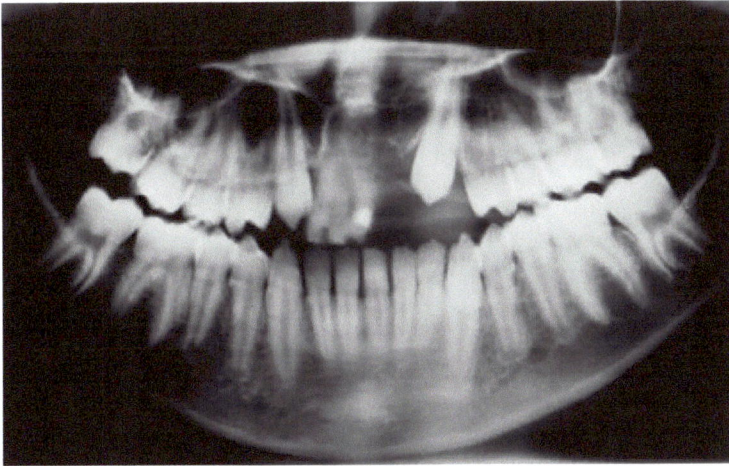

Fig. (8.8). Panoramic radiograph presenting the supernumerary mandibular incisor, of the same individual presented in Fig. (**8.7**).

ROBINOW SYNDROME

This is a rare genetic disorder, also called fetal face syndrome (Fig. **8.9**), which causes skeletal dysplasia mainly characterized by limb shortening, hyperteleorbitism and craniofacial and orodental abnormalities [15, 16]. In addition to these features, there are also reports of renal, cardiovascular and vertebral anomalies, besides hypoplastic external genitalia in males [17]. There may be variation in the severity of craniofacial characteristics, skeletal, urogenital and cardiovascular disorders. This syndrome was initially reported by Robinow in 1969 [18], on a family of 6 generations with predominant characteristic of low stature and autosomal dominant inheritance, yet later there have been reports of this syndrome with recessive inheritance pattern [17, 19].

The Robinow syndrome has thus been divided into dominant and recessive forms, considering the inheritance pattern and severity of signs and symptoms. The most severe manifestations are related to the recessive inheritance, especially concerning the musculoskeletal phenotypes [17, 19 - 21].

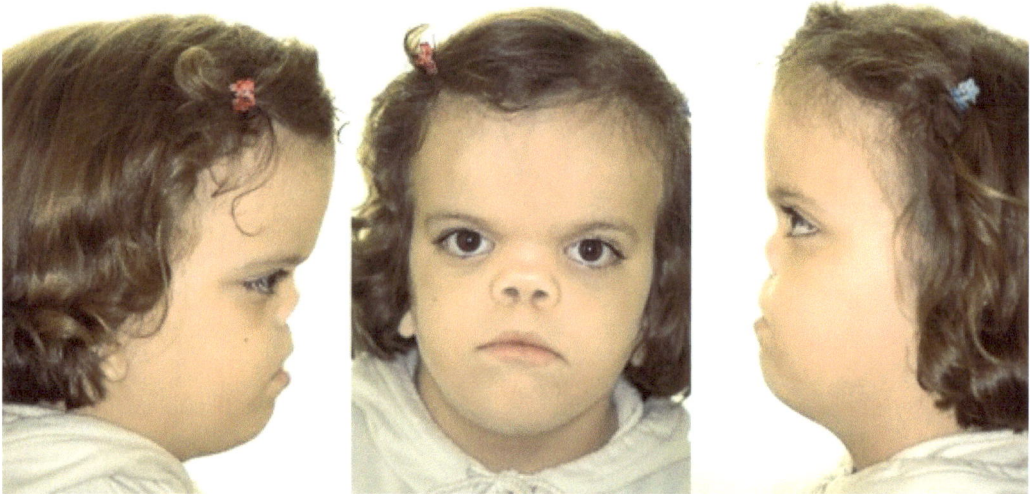

Fig. (8.9). Characteristic facial aspect in individual with Robinow syndrome.

The molecular etiology was recently described. In cases with autosomal dominant inheritance, the *WNT5A* gene has been considered a candidate in the etiology. Heterozygous mutations in this gene have been identified in some families with Robinow syndrome [17]. Conversely, mutations have been described in different positions in the *ROR2* gene in cases with recessive inheritance [15, 22].

From the standpoint of craniofacial phenotypes, the neurocranium is disproportionally wide, exhibiting dolicocephaly, prominent forehead, hypertele-orbitism, wide palpebral fissures, broad and short nose and anteverted nares [21]. The philtrum is wide in dominant cases and short in recessive cases. The ears exhibit posterior rotation. Beiraghi *et al.,* [20] reported a case series in which craniofacial dysmorphology is more severe in recessive cases.

With regard to the cognitive development, intelligence is usually normal or above average, yet some cases may exhibit intellectual disability [3, 16].

Concerning the oral aspects, there are reports of micrognathia, gingival hyperplasia, deformed alveolar ridge, supernumerary teeth, hypodontia and prolonged retention of deciduous teeth, being that some characteristics are more severe in dominant cases [17, 20, 21]. The maxillary arch presents trapezoidal shape, which may favor the occurrence of malocclusion. Cleft lip and palate are observed in 10% of cases, and the uvula is bifid or hypoplastic in 20%. There may be a small lower lip cleft and ankyloglossia [3, 16]. Dental treatment may be performed conventionally, yet including a detailed anamnesis, especially addressing the possibility of cardiovascular involvement for prevention of bacterial endocarditis. Malocclusion may be present, usually accompanied by micrognathia, and orthodontic planning should consider the analysis of bone age, which may be delayed, as well as the cardiovascular involvement.

KABUKI SYNDROME

This syndrome was initially described in two individual reports published in 1981 [23]. The clinical diagnosis of Kabuki syndrome is based on five main phenotypes: dysmorphic face, skeletal anomalies, dermatoglyphic disorders, delayed pre- and postnatal growth and intellectual disability [24 - 26]. The Kabuki syndrome received this name due to the similarity of facial aspect with the Kabuki theater makeup, a traditional Japanese theater. The facial aspects are typical and include elongated palpebral fissures, everted lateral third of the lower eyelids, thick eyelashes, ptosis, bluish sclera, sparse, wide and high-arched eyebrows, depressed nasal tip and short columella [24, 26] (Figs. **8.10** and **8.11**).

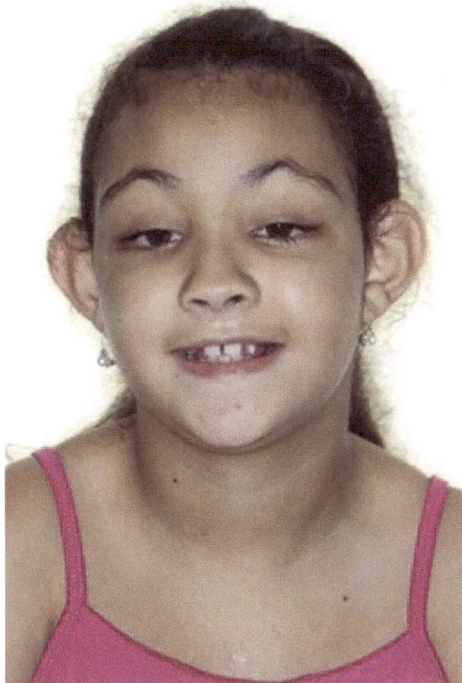

Fig. (8.10). Facial aspect in individual with Kabuki syndrome.

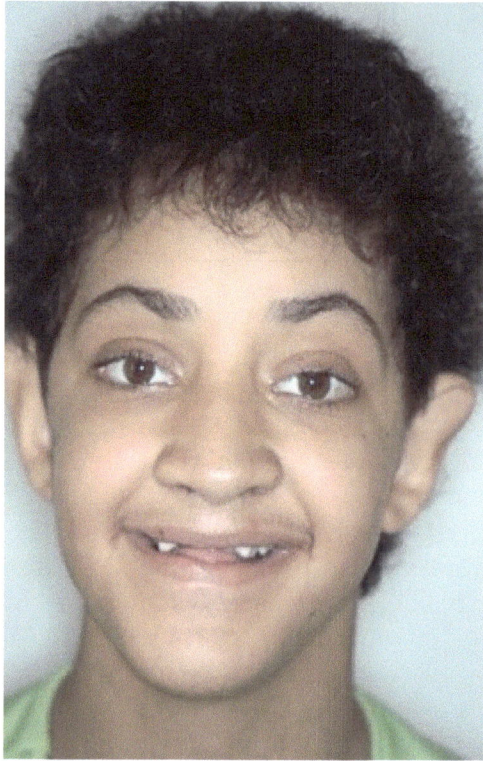

Fig. (8.11). Facial aspect in individual with Kabuki syndrome.

Analysis of affected families suggested autosomal dominant inheritance, yet most cases are sporadic. From a molecular standpoint, the etiology of the syndrome has been related to mutations in the *KMT2D* and *KDMA6* genes, and investigation of these genes is helpful to confirm the clinical diagnosis of the syndrome [24, 25].

The associated clinical findings often include cardiovascular anomalies, joint hyperextension, microcephaly, visual abnormalities [24, 28], prominent and posteriorly rotated ears, heading loss and preauricular pits. Some individuals also present intellectual disability, delayed development, hypotonia, congenital hyperthyroidism, idiopathic thrombocytopenic purpura, hemolytic anemia and susceptibility to infections [23].

The most common oral findings include dental anomalies, maxillary retrognathism, micrognathia and high-arched palate [23, 24, 27 - 31]. The reported dental anomalies include abnormalities of incisor shape [28, 32], fusion [33], hypodontia [27, 26, 30 - 32], root dilaceration [29], enamel opacity [29], delayed eruption [28], ectopic eruption of maxillary molars [32], lack of space for eruption of maxillary canines, wide pulp chamber of maxillary central incisors and permanent molars, and duplication of the apical root third in single-rooted teeth [23, 28]. Cleft lip and palate may also be observed, especially isolated cleft palate [26, 30]. In general, during dental treatment, the professional should observe the presence of systemic phenotypes that may be relevant for dental procedures, especially cardiovascular disorders, considering the need of cardiological evaluation in an interdisciplinary approach to define the need of antibiotic prophylaxis for prevention of bacterial endocarditis for dental treatment. The cognitive development of the individual should be assessed to analyze the possibility of patient compliance with dental and orthodontic treatment, which may be needed due to the skeletal alterations of the middle facial third that are characteristic of the syndrome.

CORNELIA DE LANGE SYNDROME

This is considered a rare syndrome, whose phenotype includes low birth weight, short stature and craniofacial alterations [34]. Important characteristics for differential diagnosis are the typical facial phenotype, delayed pre- and postnatal growth, limb abnormalities, especially affecting the upper limbs, and disturbances in cognitive development, with variable cases of intellectual disability (moderate to severe) and learning difficulties, even though there are reports of individuals with normal intelligence [34 - 38]. The characteristic facies of the syndrome includes low hairline, synophrys, anteverted nares and maxillary prognathism.

Even though the genetic/molecular etiology is still under investigation, 10% of cases present chromosomal alterations at the chromosome region 3q 26:2-q23. A higher percentage of cases present mutations in the *NIBPL, SMC1A, SMC3, HDAC8* and *RAD21* genes [34 - 36, 39 - 41].

Other associated phenotypes are microcephaly or brachycephaly, low-set ears, hearing loss, long and curved eyelashes and depressed nasal tip [40]. Systemically, there may be congenital cardiac defect, congenital diaphragmatic hernia, hypoplastic nipples, gastroesophageal reflux, predisposition to aspiration pneumonia, genitourinary anomalies, ophthalmological disorders (ptosis, nystagmus and myopia), cryptorchidism and genital hypoplasia in males [40, 42]. The limb involvement includes limited elbow extension, radial head displacement, single palmar crease, clinodactyly of the fifth finger, oligodactyly and syndactyly of the second and third toes [37].

In addition to maxillary prognathism and micrognathia, there are reports of thin upper lip, downslanting lip commissures, high-arched palate, cleft lip and palate, multiple diastemas and delayed tooth eruption [37, 40]. The oral findings reported by Sandhu *et al.,* [34] were macroglossia, high-arched palate, enlarged tonsils and excessive salivation. In case of severe cognitive involvement, the possibility of compliance for outpatient dental care should be assessed, with utilization of behavior management techniques.

MOEBIUS SYNDROME

The Moebius syndrome is a neurological alteration characterized by congenital paralysis of the VII cranial nerve (facial) (Fig. **8.12**) also affecting the lateral eye movement. It is often accompanied by dysfunction of other cranial nerves (II, IV, V, VI, VIII, IX, X and XII). Other associated clinical characteristics include orofacial alterations, limb malformation and hearing loss, and some cases are also diagnosed with autism spectrum disorder [43, 44]. Besides the involvement of cranial nerves, there may be peripheral neuropathy, arthrogryposis, digit contraction, strabismus and hypogonadism. There are also reports of dysphagia and respiratory problems [45]. Intellectual disability of variable extent may be observed in some cases.

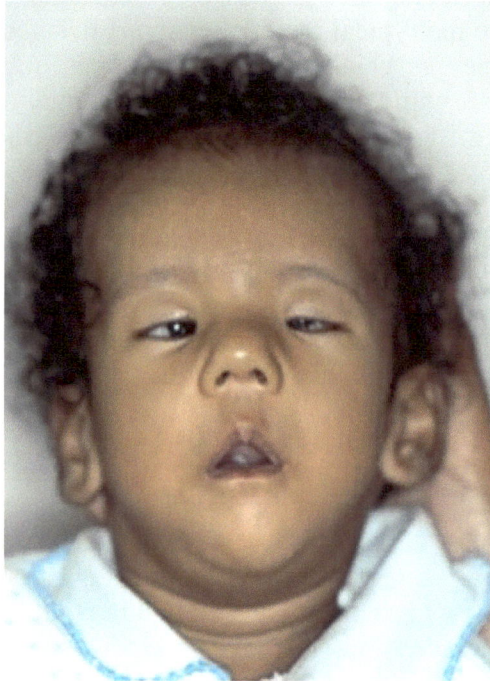

Fig. (8.12). Typical facial aspect in individual with Moebius syndrome.

Most cases are sporadic, yet there are reports of familial recurrence, which presented autosomal dominant, autosomal recessive and X-linked recessive inheritance patterns [46, 47]. In cytogenetic studies, the syndrome has been related with chromosomes 13 and 10 [46]. Except for mutations in the *HOXA1*

(MIM 142955) or *TUBB3* (MIM 602661) genes, which cause an atypical type of Moebius syndrome, the genetic etiology is not fully elucidated [44]. Recently, Tomas-Roca *et al.,* [48] suggested that both environmental intrauterine and genetic factors would be involved in the etiology and pathogenesis of the syndrome. The teratogenic environmental factors include the utilization of medications (misoprostol) and drugs (cocaine) [43, 46, 48].

The craniofacial alterations include reports of micrognathia, high-arched palate, cleft palate and tooth abnormalities [43, 46, 47]. A study conducted on 12 individuals with Moebius syndrome to investigate the oral characteristics [49] observed upper lip hypoplasia, microstomia, downslanting lip commissures, mandibular hypoplasia, high-arched palate and open bite. There are reports of tongue hypotonia, fissures, atrophy and ankyloglossia [49], as well as hypodontia of deciduous and permanent teeth [50].

Due to the lack of facial expression, during dental treatment the professional should always check the anesthesia, since the individual will be unable to manifest in case of pain. The lack of support to the lower lip should also be considered during treatment, since the individual may present excessive salivation, which may lead to angular cheilitis [43]. During outpatient dental care the professional should also be attentive to the constant control of salivation and keep the individual as seated as possible, to avoid choking. Microstomia is another feature that may complicate dental treatment [43], since the individual presented limited mouth opening for accomplishment of procedures. In this case, short treatment sessions should be planned, as well as the utilization of adapted mouth openers. Affected individuals may also present temporomandibular dysfunction with severe reduction of joint movement, which should also be considered during dental treatment [51].

CONFLICT OF INTEREST

The author (editor) declares no conflict of interest, financial or otherwise.

ACKNOWLEDGEMENTS

Declared none.

REFERENCES

[1]   Dainezi VB, Neves LT, da Silva Dalben G, Gomide MR. Tooth abnormalities and occlusal disorders in individuals with frontonasal dysplasia. Cleft Palate Craniofac J 2017; 54(3): 304-8.
[http://dx.doi.org/10.1597/15-286] [PMID: 26882026]

[2]   McKusick VA. Frontonasal dysplasia 1; FND1. Available at: http://omim.org/entry/136760

[3] Gorlin RJ, Cohen MM Junior, Levin LS. Syndromes with unusual facies: well-known syndromes. In: Gorlin RJ, Cohen MM, Hennekam RC, Eds. Syndromes of the head and neck New York. Oxford 1990; pp. 785-827.

[4] McKusick VA. Craniofrontonasal syndrome; CFNS. Available at: http://omim.org/entry/304110

[5] Twigg SR, Kan R, Babbs C, *et al.* Mutations of ephrin-B1 (EFNB1), a marker of tissue boundary formation, cause craniofrontonasal syndrome. Proc Natl Acad Sci USA 2004; 101(23): 8652-7. [http://dx.doi.org/10.1073/pnas.0402819101] [PMID: 15166289]

[6] Wieland I, Jakubiczka S, Muschke P, *et al.* Mutations of the ephrin-B1 gene cause craniofrontonasal syndrome. Am J Hum Genet 2004; 74(6): 1209-15. [http://dx.doi.org/10.1086/421532] [PMID: 15124102]

[7] Gollop TR. Fronto-facio-nasal dysostosis - a new autosomal recessive syndrome. Am J Med Genet 1981; 10(4): 409-12. [http://dx.doi.org/10.1002/ajmg.1320100415] [PMID: 7332033]

[8] McKusick VA. Frontofacionasal dysplasia. Available at: http://omim.org/entry/229400

[9] Richieri-Costa A, Colletto GM, Gollop TR, Masiero D. A previously undescribed autosomal recessive multiple congenital anomalies/mental retardation (MCA/MR) syndrome with fronto-nasal dysostosis, cleft lip/palate, limb hypoplasia, and postaxial poly-syndactyly: acro-fronto-facio-nasal dysostosis syndrome. Am J Med Genet 1985; 20(4): 631-8. [http://dx.doi.org/10.1002/ajmg.1320200409] [PMID: 2986457]

[10] Naguib KK. Hypertelorism, proptosis, ptosis, polysyndactyly, hypospadias and normal height in 3 sibs: a new syndrome? Am J Med Genet 1988; 29(1): 35-41. [http://dx.doi.org/10.1002/ajmg.1320290105] [PMID: 2830788]

[11] Chaabouni M, Maazoul F, Ben Hamida A, Berhouma M, Marrakchi Z, Chaabouni H. Autosomal recessive acro-fronto-facio-nasal dysostosis associated with genitourinary anomalies: a third case report. Am J Med Genet A 2008; 146A(14): 1825-7. [http://dx.doi.org/10.1002/ajmg.a.32349] [PMID: 18553510]

[12] McKusick VA. Opitz GBBB syndrome 1, type I; GBBB1. Available at: http://omim.org/entry/300000 2003e.

[13] Brooks JK, Leonard CO, Coccaro PJ Jr. Opitz (BBB/G) syndrome: oral manifestations. Am J Med Genet 1992; 43(3): 595-601. [http://dx.doi.org/10.1002/ajmg.1320430318] [PMID: 1605255]

[14] da Silva Dalben G, Richieri-Costa A, de Assis Taveira LA. Tooth abnormalities and soft tissue alterations in patients with G/BBB syndrome. Oral Dis 2008; 14(8): 747-53. [http://dx.doi.org/10.1111/j.1601-0825.2008.01457.x] [PMID: 18627501]

[15] Aglan M, Amr K, Ismail S, *et al.* Clinical and molecular characterization of seven Egyptian families with autosomal recessive robinow syndrome: Identification of four novel ROR2 gene mutations. Am J Med Genet A 2015; 167A(12): 3054-61. [http://dx.doi.org/10.1002/ajmg.a.37287] [PMID: 26284319]

[16] McKusick VA. Robinow syndrome, autosomal dominant 1; DRS1. Available at: http://omim.org/entry/180700 1999c.

[17] Roifman M, Marcelis CL, Paton T, *et al. De novo* WNT5A-associated autosomal dominant Robinow syndrome suggests specificity of genotype and phenotype. Clin Genet 2015; 87(1): 34-41. [http://dx.doi.org/10.1111/cge.12401] [PMID: 24716670]

[18] Robinow M, Silverman FN, Smith HD. A newly recognized dwarfing syndrome. Am J Dis Child 1969; 117(6): 645-51. [PMID: 5771504]

[19] Kantaputra PN, Gorlin RJ, Ukarapol N, Unachak K, Sudasna J. Robinow (fetal face) syndrome: report

of a boy with dominant type and an infant with recessive type. Am J Med Genet 1999; 84(1): 1-7.
[http://dx.doi.org/10.1002/(SICI)1096-8628(19990507)84:1<1::AID-AJMG1>3.0.CO;2-C] [PMID: 10213037]

[20]   Beiraghi S, Leon-Salazar V, Larson BE, *et al.* Craniofacial and intraoral phenotype of Robinow syndrome forms. Clin Genet 2011; 80(1): 15-24.
[http://dx.doi.org/10.1111/j.1399-0004.2011.01683.x] [PMID: 21496006]

[21]   Mazzeu JF, Pardono E, Vianna-Morgante AM, *et al.* Clinical characterization of autosomal dominant and recessive variants of Robinow syndrome. Am J Med Genet A 2007; 143(4): 320-5.
[http://dx.doi.org/10.1002/ajmg.a.31592] [PMID: 17256787]

[22]   Tamhankar PM, Vasudevan L, Kondurkar S, *et al.* Identification of novel ROR2 gene mutations in Indian children with Robinow syndrome. J Clin Res Pediatr Endocrinol 2014; 6(2): 79-83.
[http://dx.doi.org/10.4274/jcrpe.1233] [PMID: 24932600]

[23]   McKusick VA. Kabuki syndrome 1; Kabuk1. Available at: http://omim.org/entry/147920 2003e.

[24]   Dentici ML, Di Pede A, Lepri FR, *et al.* Kabuki syndrome: clinical and molecular diagnosis in the first year of life. Arch Dis Child 2015; 100(2): 158-64.
[http://dx.doi.org/10.1136/archdischild-2013-305858] [PMID: 25281733]

[25]   Liu S, Hong X, Shen C, *et al.* Kabuki syndrome: a Chinese case series and systematic review of the spectrum of mutations. BMC Med Genet 2015; 16: 26.
[http://dx.doi.org/10.1186/s12881-015-0171-4] [PMID: 25896430]

[26]   Pinto LC. Caracterização odontológica dos indivíduos com síndrome de Kabuki: estudo clínico e radiográfico retrospectivo [thesis]; Bauru 2014.

[27]   Matsune K, Shimizu T, Tohma T, Asada Y, Ohashi H, Maeda T. Craniofacial and dental characteristics of Kabuki syndrome. Am J Med Genet 2001; 98(2): 185-90.
[http://dx.doi.org/10.1002/1096-8628(20010115)98:2<185::AID-AJMG1029>3.0.CO;2-M] [PMID: 11223856]

[28]   Petzold D, Kratzsch E, Opitz Ch, Tinschert S. The Kabuki syndrome: four patients with oral abnormalities. Eur J Orthod 2003; 25(1): 13-9.
[http://dx.doi.org/10.1093/ejo/25.1.13] [PMID: 12608719]

[29]   do Prado Sobral S, Leite AF, Figueiredo PT, *et al.* Craniofacial and dental features in kabuki syndrome patients. Cleft Palate Craniofac J 2013; 50(4): 440-7.
[http://dx.doi.org/10.1597/11-052] [PMID: 22023252]

[30]   Teixeira CS, Silva CR, Honjo RS, Bertola DR, Albano LM, Kim CA. Dental evaluation of Kabuki syndrome patients. Cleft Palate Craniofac J 2009; 46(6): 668-73.
[http://dx.doi.org/10.1597/08-077.1] [PMID: 19860501]

[31]   Tuna EB, Marşan G, Gençay K, Seymen F. Craniofacial and dental characteristics of Kabuki syndrome: nine years cephalometric follow-up. J Clin Pediatr Dent 2012; 36(4): 393-400.
[http://dx.doi.org/10.17796/jcpd.36.4.u021164272805116] [PMID: 23019839]

[32]   Mhanni AA, Cross HG, Chudley AE. Kabuki syndrome: description of dental findings in 8 patients. Clin Genet 1999; 56(2): 154-7.
[http://dx.doi.org/10.1034/j.1399-0004.1999.560211.x] [PMID: 10517254]

[33]   dos Santos BM, Ribeiro RR, Stuani AS, de Paula e Silva FW, de Queiroz AM. Kabuki make-up (Niikawa-Kuroki) syndrome: dental and craniofacial findings in a Brazilian child. Braz Dent J 2006; 17(3): 249-54.
[http://dx.doi.org/10.1590/S0103-64402006000300014] [PMID: 17262134]

[34]   Sandhu M, Nagpal M, Gulia S, Sachdev V. Dental management of cornelia de lange syndrome: a rare case report. J Clin Diagn Res 2015; 9(2): ZD12-4.
[PMID: 25859533]

[35]   Deardorff MA, Kaur M, Yaeger D, *et al.* Mutations in cohesin complex members SMC3 and SMC1A cause a mild variant of cornelia de Lange syndrome with predominant mental retardation. Am J Hum Genet 2007; 80(3): 485-94.
[http://dx.doi.org/10.1086/511888] [PMID: 17273969]

[36]   Gil-Rodríguez MC, Deardorff MA, Ansari M, *et al. De novo* heterozygous mutations in SMC3 cause a range of Cornelia de Lange syndrome-overlapping phenotypes. Hum Mutat 2015; 36(4): 454-62.
[http://dx.doi.org/10.1002/humu.22761] [PMID: 25655089]

[37]   McKusick VA. Cornelia de Lange syndrome 1; CDL1. Available at: http://omim.org/entry/122470 2003b.

[38]   Saal HM, Samango-Sprouse CA, Rodnan LA, Rosenbaum KN, Custer DA. Brachmann-de Lange syndrome with normal IQ. Am J Med Genet 1993; 47(7): 995-8.
[http://dx.doi.org/10.1002/ajmg.1320470711] [PMID: 8291543]

[39]   Hoppman-Chaney N, Jang JS, Jen J, Babovic-Vuksanovic D, Hodge JC. In-frame multi-exon deletion of SMC1A in a severely affected female with Cornelia de Lange Syndrome. Am J Med Genet A 2012; 158A(1): 193-8.
[http://dx.doi.org/10.1002/ajmg.a.34360] [PMID: 22106055]

[40]   Pié J, Gil-Rodríguez MC, Ciero M, *et al.* Mutations and variants in the cohesion factor genes NIPBL, SMC1A, and SMC3 in a cohort of 30 unrelated patients with Cornelia de Lange syndrome. Am J Med Genet A 2010; 152A(4): 924-9.
[http://dx.doi.org/10.1002/ajmg.a.33348] [PMID: 20358602]

[41]   Yuan B, Pehlivan D, Karaca E, *et al.* Global transcriptional disturbances underlie Cornelia de Lange syndrome and related phenotypes. J Clin Invest 2015; 125(2): 636-51.
[http://dx.doi.org/10.1172/JCI77435] [PMID: 25574841]

[42]   Levin AV, Seidman DJ, Nelson LB, Jackson LG. Ophthalmologic findings in the Cornelia de Lange syndrome. J Pediatr Ophthalmol Strabismus 1990; 27(2): 94-102.
[PMID: 2348318]

[43]   Pradhan A, Gryst M. Atraumatic restorative technique: case report on dental management of a patient with Moebius syndrome. Aust Dent J 2015; 60(2): 255-9.
[http://dx.doi.org/10.1111/adj.12319] [PMID: 25989267]

[44]   Webb BD, Shaaban S, Gaspar H, *et al.* HOXB1 founder mutation in humans recapitulates the phenotype of Hoxb1-/- mice. Am J Hum Genet 2012; 91(1): 171-9.
[http://dx.doi.org/10.1016/j.ajhg.2012.05.018] [PMID: 22770981]

[45]   Matsui K, Kataoka A, Yamamoto A, *et al.* Clinical characteristics and outcomes of Möbius syndrome in a children's hospital. Pediatr Neurol 2014; 51(6): 781-9.
[http://dx.doi.org/10.1016/j.pediatrneurol.2014.08.011] [PMID: 25306435]

[46]   Guedes ZC. Möbius syndrome: misoprostol use and speech and language characteristics. Int Arch Otorhinolaryngol 2014; 18(3): 239-43.
[http://dx.doi.org/10.1055/s-0033-1363466] [PMID: 25992099]

[47]   Verzijl HT, van der Zwaag B, Cruysberg JR, Padberg GW. Möbius syndrome redefined: a syndrome of rhombencephalic maldevelopment. Neurology 2003; 61(3): 327-33.
[http://dx.doi.org/10.1212/01.WNL.0000076484.91275.CD] [PMID: 12913192]

[48]   Tomas-Roca L, Tsaalbi-Shtylik A, Jansen JG, *et al. De novo* mutations in *PLXND1* and *REV3L* cause Möbius syndrome. Nat Commun 2015; 6: 7199.
[http://dx.doi.org/10.1038/ncomms8199] [PMID: 26068067]

[49]   De Serpa Pinto MV, De Magalhães MH, Nunes FD. Moebius syndrome with oral involvement. Int J Paediatr Dent 2002; 12(6): 446-9.
[http://dx.doi.org/10.1046/j.1365-263X.2002.00402.x] [PMID: 12452989]

[50]   Rizos M, Negrón RJ, Serman N. Möbius syndrome with dental involvement: a case report and literature review. Cleft Palate Craniofac J 1998; 35(3): 262-8.
[http://dx.doi.org/10.1597/1545-1569(1998)035<0262:MBSWDI>2.3.CO;2] [PMID: 9603562]

[51]   Di Blasio A, Cassi D, Di Blasio C, Gandolfini M. Temporomandibular joint dysfunction in Moebius syndrome. Eur J Paediatr Dent 2013; 14(4): 295-8.
[PMID: 24313581]

CHAPTER 9

Surgical Treatment in Craniofacial Malformations: Distraction Osteogenesis

Cristiano Tonello*, Adriano Porto Peixoto*, Maurício Mitsuru Yoshida*, Michele Madeira Brandão*, Melissa Zattoni Antoneli** and Nivaldo Alonso**

Hospital for Rehabilitation of Craniofacial Anomalies, University of São Paulo, Brazil

Abstract: Distraction Osteogenesis (DO), a procedure used for correction of large hypoplasia of facial segments, is a surgical technique that induces new bone formation by gradual separation of two bone surfaces osteotomized by a mechanical device called distractor; the principles of this surgery were initially designed by the Russian orthopedist Gavriil Ilizarov in 1951. Different pathological conditions, mostly syndromic, may present craniofacial deformities that may not be functionally and esthetically corrected by conventional treatment methods. Some examples include the mandibular hypoplasias (Pierre Robin sequence, Oculoauriculovertebral spectrum (OAVS), Treacher Collins syndrome, temporomandibular joint ankylosis, hypoplasia of the midface (common finding in individuals with syndromic craniosynostosis, such as the Apert, Crouzon, Pfeiffer, Muenke and Saethre-Chotzen syndromes). Even though DO is the method of excellence for the treatment of large hypoplasias, it should only be used when a large dentofacial deformity cannot be corrected by conventional orthognathic surgery, which may be used to refine the results achieved by DO in a second auxiliary stage.

Keywords: Congenital anomalies, Distraction osteogenesis, Orthodontics.

Distraction osteogenesis is characterized as a dynamic process, which comprises elongation of the facial skeleton and adjacent soft tissues, obtained by gradual

---

* **Corresponding author Cristiano Tonello:** Hospital for Rehabilitation of Craniofacial Anomalies, University of São Paulo, Bauru, Brazil; Tel/Fax: +55 14 3235-8000; E-mail: cristianotonello@hotmail.com; cristianotonello@usp.br
* **Adriano Porto Peixoto:** Hospital for Rehabilitation of Craniofacial Anomalies, University of São Paulo, Bauru, Brazil; Tel/Fax: +55 14 3235-8000; E-mail: adrianoporto@usp.br
* **Maurício Mitsuru Yoshida:** Santa Marcelina Hospital, São Paulo, Brazil; Tel/Fax: +55 11 2070-6000; E-mail: mauricio_yoshida@uol.com.br
* **Michele Madeira Brandão:** Hospital for Rehabilitation of Craniofacial Anomalies, University of São Paulo, Bauru, Brazil; Tel/Fax: +55 14 3235-8000; E-mail: luchele@uol.com.br
** **Melissa Zattoni Antoneli:** Hospital for Rehabilitation of Craniofacial Anomalies, University of São Paulo, Bauru, Brazil; Tel/Fax: +55 14 3235-8000; E-mail: melfono@usp.br
** **Nivaldo Alonso:** Medical School and Hospital for Rehabilitation of Craniofacial Anomalies, University of São Paulo, Bauru, Brazil; Tel/Fax: +55 11 3061-7000; E-mail: nivalonso@gmail.com

traction applied on two osteotomized bone surfaces by a mechanical device called distractor (Fig. **9.1**).

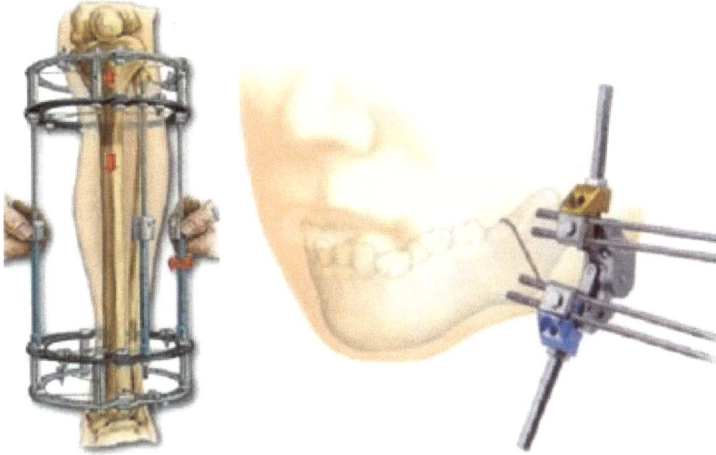

Fig. (9.1). Distractors for mandible and long bone of the leg. Similar principles applied for bone elongation. Source: modified from Hong PA. Clinical narrative review of mandibular distraction osteogenesis in neonates with Pierre Robin sequence. Int J Pediatr Otorhinolaryngol 2011;75(8):985-91.

A sequence of adaptive changes, as observed in the bone tissue, also occurs in the soft tissues. The gradual elongation of these structures minimizes the potential of relapse posed by the resistance of soft tissues in large bone displacements [1 - 4].

DISTRACTION OSTEOGENESIS IN CRANIOFACIAL MALFORMATIONS

1. Principles and Stages

In 1951 the Russian orthopedist Gavriil Ilizarov initiated a series of experimental and clinical studies, establishing the principles of the bone elongation method [1, 3].

Its important contribution was related to the understanding of biological events involved in the process of bone elongation. Distraction osteogenesis, named as such by Ilizarov, is based on the fact that gradual and sustained traction, applied on a living tissue, creates a tension that stimulates tissue regeneration and growth by activating the cellular proliferative and biosynthetic functions.

The success achieved in correcting several types of skeletal deformities by elongation of endochondral bones led to wide acceptance of this method, so as these principles were then also applied on the craniofacial segment.

The first applications of distraction in humans were conducted by McCarthy [5] in 1992, who described the elongation of hypoplastic mandibles, and Cohen *et al.*, [6], who described the first report of utilization of DO to correct deformities of the midface in 1995.

From a didactic standpoint, distraction osteogenesis may be divided in four stages:

- Formation of blood clot;
- Formation of fibrous callus (elongation occurs on the fibrous callus);
- Bone calcification;
- Remodeled newly formed bone.

2. Clinical Indications

Different pathological conditions, mostly syndromic, are accompanied by craniofacial deformities that may not be esthetically and functionally corrected by conventional treatment methods. Therefore, its clinical application is essentially based on correction of large hypoplasias of the facial segments, especially mandibular hypoplasia and hypoplasias of the midface [7].

2.1. Mandibular Hypoplasias

Mandibular growth disorders occur in three main situations:

a. Pierre Robin sequence
b. Oculoauriculovertebral spectrum (OAVS)
c. Treacher Collins syndrome

These disorders may affect the mandible unilaterally or bilaterally. The involvement of other anatomical structures as the maxilla, zygoma, muscles of mastication and adjacent soft tissues further complicates the treatment of these individuals.

The common embryonic origin of the mandible and adjacent structures as the ear, for example, explain the findings of unilateral mandibular hypoplasia associated with ipsilateral microtia (ear malformation), as in the case of oculoauriculovertebral spectrum (Fig. **9.2**).

The Pruzansky classification is the most used system for classification of mandibular hypoplasia, scoring four different types of involvement (Fig. **9.3**):

- Type I or Pruzansky I: mandible with normal anatomy, yet with reduced size;
- Type II or Pruzansky II: hypoplastic mandible associated with malformation of

the condyle and coronoid process;

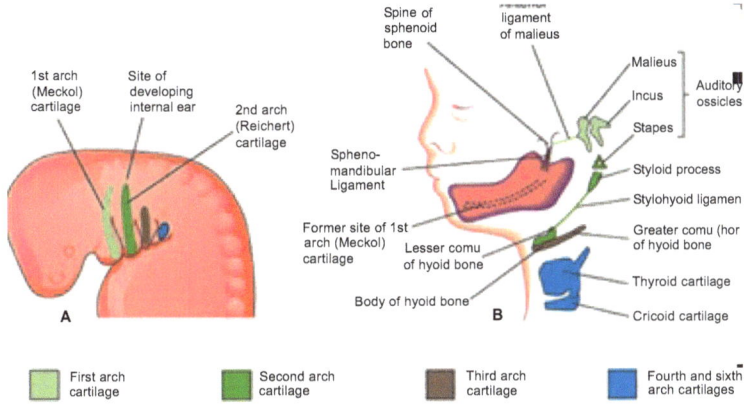

Fig. (9.2). Embryonic origin of the mandible and ear and adjacent structures (Moore and Persaud 1998, 2008).

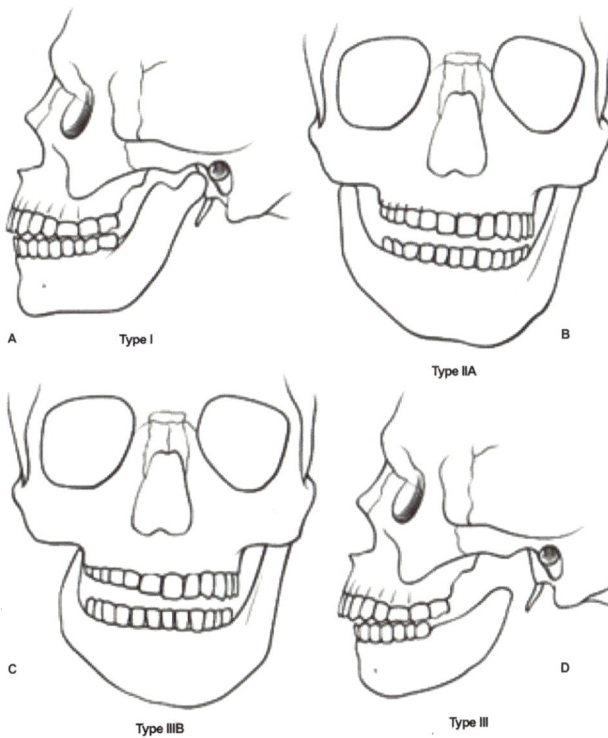

Fig. (9.3). Pruzansky classification. Source: Coccaro PJ, Pruzansky S. Longitudinal study of skeletal and soft tissue profile in children with unilateral cleft lip and cleft palate. Cleft Palate J. 1965;45:1-12.

Mulliken and Kaban later divided this group into IIA and IIB [8]:

- Type IIA: hypoplastic mandible with hypoplastic and malformed condyle, yet the condyle head maintains its spatial relationship with the glenoid cavity, similar to the contralateral side;
- Type IIB: severe condylar malformation and hypoplasia, displaced from the sagittal plane and without contact with the glenoid cavity (which is also altered in these individuals). These individuals often present restricted joint function;
- Type III or Pruzansky III: severely hypoplastic mandible with absence of the condyle, ramus, coronoid process and glenoid fossa.

2.1.a) Pierre Robin Sequence

Commonly referred to as Pierre Robin syndrome, its correct name highlights the sequence of embryonic events that cause this clinical condition (Fig. **9.4**).

The Pierre Robin sequence (PRS) is defined by the following triad [9, 10]:

- micrognathia;
- glossoptosis (retropositioning of the tongue base); and
- respiratory discomfort associated with cleft palate in most cases.

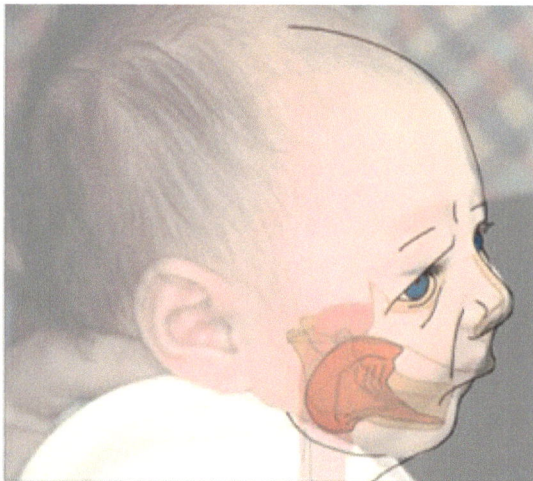

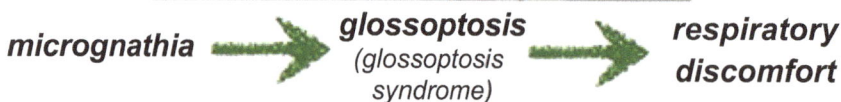

micrognathia ➡ **glossoptosis** *(glossoptosis syndrome)* ➡ **respiratory discomfort**

Fig. (9.4). Triad that characterizes the Pierre Robin sequence. Source: modified from Evans KN, Sie KC, Hopper RA, Glass RP, Hing AV, Cunningham ML. Robin Sequence: from diagnosis to development of an effective management plan. Pediatrics 2011;127:936-48.

The mandibular hypoplasia, called micrognathia, may be considered the initial embryonic event that triggers the tongue retropositioning (glossoptosis) and consequent obstruction of the upper airway, due to collapse of the tongue over the posterior pharyngeal wall in newborns. In most cases the retropositioned tongue, secondary to mandibular hypoplasia, prevents fusion of the palatal shelves in the midline during the period of embryonic formation of the palate. For this reason, 60 to 90% of individuals with PRS present U-shaped cleft of the soft palate, due to the configuration of tongue interposition on the fusion of palatal shelves and palate formation [11].

Even though most children with micrognathia or PRS are asymptomatic or may be treated only by conservative measures, some individuals present significant respiratory and swallowing impairment, requiring surgical intervention.

The conservative therapy varies from prone positioning of the newborn, up to utilization of nasopharyngeal cannulas and CPAP (*continuous positive airway pressure*) [12].

However, severe obstruction of the upper airway secondary to PRS that do not respond to conservative treatment require urgent medical assistance. Traditionally, tracheostomy has been the most effective and definitive therapeutic option for these individuals. However, tracheostomy is often associated with morbidity, high cost and occasional mortality.

Thus, distraction osteogenesis of the mandible is an alternative method to traditional techniques for airway management in these individuals, and may replace the indication for tracheostomy to allow upper airway permeability. The gradual mandibular elongation promotes anteriorization of the tongue base, thus allowing opening of the posterior airway (Fig. **9.5**).

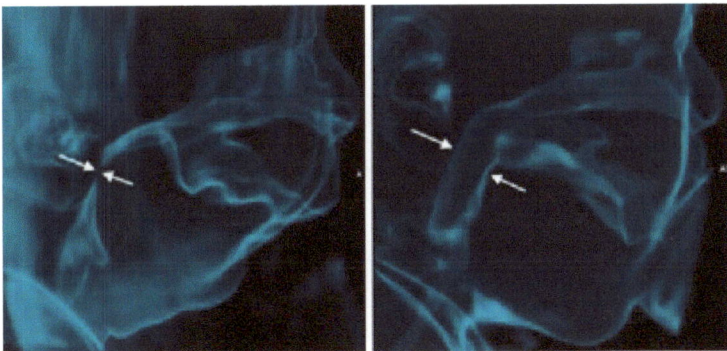

Fig. (9.5). Three-dimensional reconstruction of the airway in individual submitted to mandibular distraction osteogenesis with marked increase of the posterior airway. Source: Jarrahy R. Controversies in the management of neonatal micrognathia: to distract or not to distract. that is the question. J Craniofac Surg 2012;23(1):243-9.

For further information on Robin sequence, please refer to Chapter 5.

2.1.b) Oculoauriculovertebral Spectrum

Oculoauriculovertebral spectrum is considered the most common craniofacial anomaly after cleft lip and palate, affecting 1 in every 4,000 to 5,600 livebirths [13, 14]. This congenital condition primarily affects structures derived from the first and second pharyngeal arches as the ears, mandible and facial soft tissues [15].

These structures are affected bilaterally yet to variable extents, leading to an asymmetrical aspect of the face [16]. The etiology and pathogenesis are still unknown [15].

The first and second pharyngeal arches, which are composed of mesenchymal cells derived from mesodermal cells and cranial neural crest cells, give rise to a variety of facial structures that include skeletal, muscular and neural components, by a complex network of signals that is not fully elucidated [17]. Alterations in these signaling pathways constitute a potential source of developmental facial abnormalities. Thus, the manifestations and severity of defects depend on the expression and activation of genes and proteins during facial development [17].

The term oculoauriculovertebral spectrum (OAVS) was suggested by Cohen *et al.*, [18] to represent the different combinations of mandibular, ear, ocular and vertebral anomalies.

Other terms often employed in cases involving different combinations of these findings are oculoauriculovertebral dysplasia (OAVD), Goldenhar syndrome (GS), hemifacial microsomia (HFM), otomandibular dysostosis, pharyngeal 1st and 2nd arches syndrome and craniofacial microsomia (CFM) [18 - 20].

Clinical Findings

Despite the lack of consensus about the minimum diagnostic criteria, the structures usually affected include [16]:

• mandibular condyle and ramus;
• zygomatic arch and malar bones;
• external and middle ears and temporal bone;
• facial expression muscles.

Some authors consider the presence of isolated microtia or ear or preauricular abnormalities as milder manifestations [21]. The involvement is not limited to facial structures and may be associated with cardiac, renal and skeletal abnormalities, besides other disorders [21].

Dentofacial anomalies include cleft lip and palate, high-arched palate, hypoplastic maxillary and mandibular arches, micrognathia, gingival hypertrophy, supernumerary teeth, dentin and enamel malformations, delayed tooth development, malocclusion, macrostomia, asymmetric masticatory muscles and salivary gland agenesis [22].

Treatment Objectives

The treatment objectives include the achievement of facial symmetry, functional mandibular movement, adequate occlusion and patient satisfaction [15]. Therefore, treatment should aim to:

1. create an articulation between mandible and temporal bone, when absent;
2. correct secondary maxillary deformities;
3. establish functional occlusion with esthetic improvement of the face and dentition;
4. increase the mandibular size which is malformed or hypodeveloped, with indication for mandibular distraction osteogenesis.

The treatment should be performed in stages following a predictive sequence of biological development [15].

In more severe cases, mandibular hypoplasia may lead to airway obstruction. Thus, mandibular reconstruction or mandibular distraction osteogenesis may be necessary in earlier stages.

Lip repair, associated with correction of macrostomia, and palate repair are performed respectively after 3 months and 12 months of age. If mandibular hypoplasia does not affect the respiratory pattern, it may be managed after 6 years of age, either by costochondral graft or distraction osteogenesis. Ear reconstruction with autogenous costal cartilage is indicated after 8 years of age, when the individual presents sufficient thoracic structures as donor site. Hypoplasia of facial soft tissues may be treated by serial fat grafts. Orthognathic surgery and finally rhinoplasty are indicated after craniofacial skeletal maturity, after 15 years of age.

For further information about the oculoauriculovertebral spectrum, please refer to Chapter 7.

Surgical treatment protocol for oculoauriculovertebral spectrum

AGE	SURGICAL PROCEDURE
EARLY	Correction of respiratory alteration Mandibular reconstruction with costochondral graft Mandibular distraction osteogenesis
3-6 MONTHS	Lip repair / correction of macrostomia
12 MONTHS	Palate repair
AFTER 6 YEARS	Mandibular reconstruction with costochondral graft Mandibular distraction osteogenesis
AFTER 8 YEARS	Ear reconstruction with costal cartilage Fat graft
AFTER 15 YEARS	Orthognathic surgery Rhinoplasty

Source: Protocol adopted by the Craniofacial team of HRAC/USP Bauru.

2.1.c) Treacher Collins Syndrome

The Treacher Collins, or mandibulofacial dysostosis, is an autosomal dominant disorder with variable expressivity, complete penetrance and prevalence of 1:25,000 to 1:50,000 livebirths, characterized by bilateral symmetric abnormalities of structures derived from the first and second pharyngeal arches. The first descriptions of the syndrome are assigned to Berry (1889), Treacher Collins (1900), Franceschetti and Klein (1949) [23].

Clinical Findings

The adult individual with full expression of the syndrome presents convex facial profile, prominent nasal dorsum an retruded mandible and chin.

The eyes are characterized by downslanting palpebral fissures, due to coloboma of the lower eyelids, lateral canthal dystopia and inferolateral orbital dystopia.

The external ears are absent, malformed or malpositioned, and hearing loss is impaired due to the variable degrees of hypoplasia of the external auditory canal and middle ear ossicles. The presence of cleft palate, with or without cleft lip and choanal atresia, is variable.

The most characteristic finding of the syndrome is hypoplasia of zygomatic bones, often with clefts through the arches and limited formation of residual zygomas. The mandible and maxilla are also characteristically hypoplastic, with variable effects on the temporomandibular joint and mastication muscles. Individuals usually present Angle Class II malocclusion with anterior open bite and clockwise rotation of the occlusal plane [17, 24].

Thus, these malformations of craniofacial skeleton may yield both esthetic and functional disorders. The evaluation of disturbances in respiration, mastication, speech, swallowing, and corneal exposure should be prioritized. The degree of malformations present at birth is believed to remain stable, without progression with age [24].

Treatment Objectives

Complete rehabilitation of individuals with Treacher Collins syndrome is challenging. Several facial structures are affected, which requires specific surgical procedures at adequate ages that do not preclude or affect the other necessary procedures. Thus, the standardization of surgical approaches provides a more organized and optimized treatment.

In the population of individuals with Treacher Collins syndrome, 66% of affected individuals require some intervention in the airway [25]. Thus, maintenance of adequate airway is priority in newborns with Treacher Collins syndrome [26]. Dysphagia and difficult weight gain are often primary symptoms of the airway involvement [27].

In the neonatal period, the evaluation is initiated by examination of the airway concerning the risk to obstruction due to retromicrognathia present in more severe cases. Also, individuals with Treacher Collins syndrome present reduced posterior facial height, which also contributes to restriction of the naso-oropharyngeal spaces [28]. Individuals with severe respiratory insufficiency should be submitted to tracheostomy, while mild to moderate cases may be initially treated with nasopharyngeal cannula and followed up with oximetry and clinical evaluation. Individuals not responding favorably with the cannula should be submitted to mandibular distraction osteogenesis if the pattern of obstruction observed by nasofibroscopy is favorable (Fig. **9.6**). The aim is to avoid tracheostomy, which should be indicated as the last resource for cases not responding favorably to other measures.

Choanal atresia is other malformation associated with respiratory disturbances in the neonatal period. Children with choanal atresia without signs of respiratory insufficiency may be submitted to elective surgery to correct this alteration, yet cases evolving with respiratory insufficiency should be submitted to tracheostomy.

Mandibular distraction osteogenesis aims at increasing the oropharyngeal space, which is characteristically reduced in individuals with Treacher Collins syndrome due to the mandibular size and shape. Individuals previously submitted to tracheostomy are also analyzed for planning of elective mandibular distraction to allow earlier removal of the cannula.

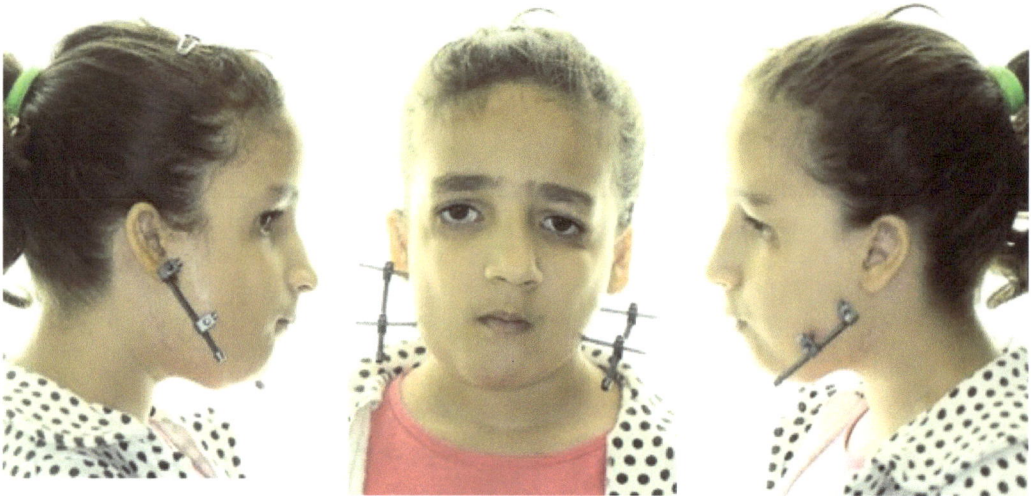

Fig. (9.6). Individual with Treacher Collins syndrome submitted to mandibular distraction osteogenesis for treatment of obstructive sleep apnea syndrome, often observed in these individuals.

After airway stabilization and nutritional adaptation, the first interventions include lip repair (after 3 months) and palate repair (after 1 year). Other procedures that may be necessary in the first year of life include correction of macrostomia and/or removal of preauricular pits.

Even though the palpebral and orbital deformities are remarkable characteristics of the syndrome, their correction should be performed later, except for individuals with inadequate palpebral occlusion with corneal exposure, who should be submitted to earlier management with transposition of musculocutaneous flap of the upper to the lower eyelid associated with lateral canthopexy. Individuals without corneal exposure may be treated concomitantly with malar reconstruction.

Malar hypoplasia is confirmed especially by the reduced interzygomatic distance and zygomatic arch length [29]. Malar reconstruction is postponed up to 6 years of age, until achievement of more complete cranio-orbito-zygomatic complex. Waitzman stated that, at 5 years of age, the cranio-orbito-zygomatic skeleton reaches more than 85% of the skeletal development of an adult [30]. The zygoma body and lateral orbit wall are anatomical regions that should be reconstructed with priority. The procedure is performed by exclusively intraoral access, using full thickness bone graft from the calvaria with rigid fixation. The procedure is associated with palpebral reconstruction with transposition of myocutaneous flap from the upper to the lower eyelid with lateral canthopexy. Even though the exclusively intraoral surgical access limits the operative field, the association with bicoronal incision classically described for bone graft achievement and reconstruction of the lateral orbit wall may compromise the temporal fascia, which will be needed later for ear reconstruction.

After 8 years of age, ear reconstruction is performed with autogenous costal cartilage in two stages, creating a cartilage framework from the costal cartilages of three ribs from the same side of the defect on the first stage, followed by elevation and coverage of the cartilage framework with temporoparietal fascia flap and split thickness cutaneous graft on the second stage.

The maxilla in individuals with Treacher Collins syndrome is significantly shorter, as well as the mandible, which is also retropositioned and presents clockwise rotation, yielding a convex facial profile with premature posterior tooth contacts and anterior open bite. Mandibular alteration is important in all components of growth with reduction of ramus vertical height, mandibular body length and mandibular body bone volume [28].

Orthognathic surgery is indicated after facial skeletal maturity, which is completed between 15 to 18 years of age. Typically, Le Fort I maxillary osteotomy is associated with sagittal mandibular osteotomy and mentoplasty. The reduced mandibular ramus height and increased antegonial incisure, combined with the need of great advancements and mandibular rotations in more severe cases, requires careful planning of sagittal osteotomy to assure sufficient bone contact after mobilization of the distal segment [28]. If mandibular deformity is more severe, with reduced mandibular ramus dimensions, vertical distraction osteogenesis of the mandibular ramus should be performed first to provide greater bone contact in sagittal osteotomy [28].

Finally, rhinoseptoplasty is performed after orthognathic surgery, with reduction of osteocartilaginous dorsum, removal of cephalic portions of inferior lateral cartilages, structuration of the nasal tip with columella strut and nasal osteotomy [31]. Soft tissue deficiencies at the malar region are treated with serial fat grafts of small volume.

Surgical treatment protocol for Treacher Collins syndrome

AGE	SURGICAL PROCEDURE
EARLY	Correction of respiratory alteration Mandibular distraction osteogenesis Correction of choanal atresia Tracheostomy Palpebral reconstruction (in case of corneal exposure)
3-6 MONTHS	Lip repair / correction of macrostomia

AGE	SURGICAL PROCEDURE
12 MONTHS	Palate repair
AFTER 6 YEARS	Malar reconstruction with autogenous bone graft from the calvaria Palpebral reconstruction + lateral canthopexy Mandibular reconstruction with costochondral graft Mandibular distraction osteogenesis
AFTER 8 YEARS	Ear reconstruction with costal cartilage Fat graft
AFTER 15 YEARS	Orthognathic surgery Rhinoplasty

Source: Thompson JT, Anderson PJ, David DJ. Treacher Collins syndrome: protocol management from birth to maturity. The Journal of craniofacial surgery. 2009;20(6):2028-35. Yoshida M, Tonello C, Alonso N. Síndrome de Treacher Collins: desafio na otimização do tratamento cirúrgico. Rev Bras Cir Craniomaxilofac. 2012;15(2):64-8

Surgical Technique

Different types of distractors were designed to achieve elongation of facial bones. These may be external, when fixated to the bone by percutaneous pins; or internal, when entirely inserted below the skin or oral mucosa, maintaining only the access to the rod for appliance activation.

The main advantage of distraction osteogenesis is the possibility of earlier treatment of bone deformities, besides allowing expansion of adjacent soft tissues, which contributes to the stability of reconstruction with consequent reduction in the relapse risk [32].

The operative technique comprises incision of 3 to 5 cm along the oblique line of the mandibular ramus in the oral mucosa, under general anesthesia. Subperiosteal dissection is performed to expose the gonial angle and adjacent area of the ascending ramus. Following, the site of corticotomy is defined at the junction between angle and ascending ramus (according to the mandibular deformity, corticotomy may be more anterior or vertical). Using a reciprocating saw, corticotomy is performed at the lateral aspect of the mandible, including the entire thickness of external cortical plate, in oblique direction from the free mandibular margin up to the gonial angle. Following, internal corticotomy is performed at the region of the gonial angle, taking care to avoid damage to the inferior alveolar nerve, located between the two cortical plates. Titanium rods (in external distractors) are introduced percutaneously, 4 to 5 mm in proximal position and distal to the corticotomy; in internal distractors, they are fixated directly into the bone using titanium screws. After adequate positioning of distractors, they are activated intraoperatively to check the efficacy of distraction [33, 34]. If resistance is felt, corticotomy should be revised with auxiliary utilization of chisels to complement the osteotomy, especially at the internal aspect (Fig. **9.7**).

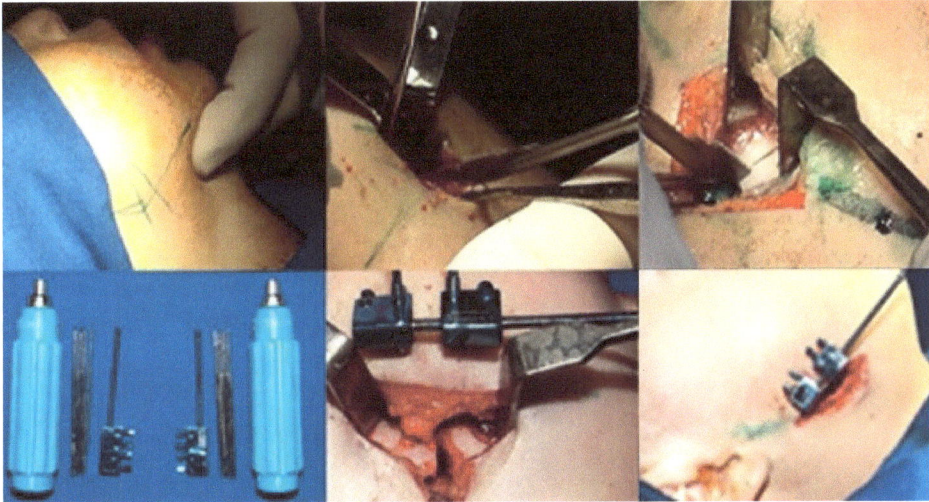

Fig. (9.7). Sequence of photographs demonstrating the different surgical stages for placement of external mandibular distraction and immediate postoperative aspect.

Defining the distraction vector is a critical decision [33, 35, 36]. Corticotomy and the position of rods or screws determine the distraction vector. According to the characteristics of mandibular hypoplasia, the distraction vector is different for each case [33, 34].

As all surgical procedures, distraction osteogenesis also involves risks of accidents, with prevalence of 2.5 to 35% [37]. The most frequent events include resistance upon distractor activation, pain at the regenerating bone site, infection, loss of distractor stability, premature consolidation, and others [37].

For further information about Treachery Collins syndrome, please refer to Chapter 7.

2.2. Hypoplasia of the Midface

Hypoplasia of the Midface is a common finding in individuals with syndromic craniosynostosis. The craniosynostosis comprises premature fusion of one or more cranial sutures [38]. Craniosynostoses may be classified as non-syndromic, when there is involvement only of cranial sutures, and syndromic, when associated with other anomalies, such as craniofacial deformities [39 - 41].

Even though the non-syndromic craniosynostoses account for most cases, with approximate prevalence of 1:2,000, so far more than 150 syndromes have been associated with these conditions [42]. Among the syndromic craniosynostoses, the Apert and Crouzon syndromes (prevalence 1:60,000 livebirths), Pfeiffer, Muenke and Saethre-Chotzen syndromes are the commonest [43].

Below, notice the two main syndromes (Fig. **9.8**) associated with hypoplasia of the midface:

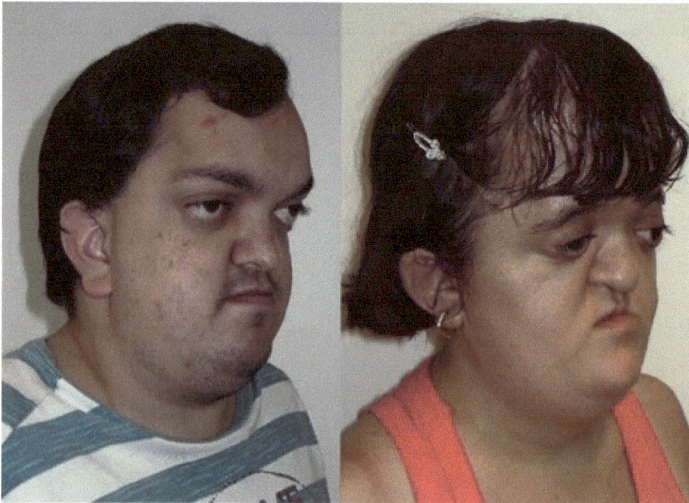

Fig. (9.8). Individual with marked retrusion of the midface, yet with different characteristics oi in the Crouzon and Apert syndromes, respectively.

Crouzon Syndrome

This is characterized by craniosynostosis, exorbitism and retruded midface, with autosomal dominant inheritance. There is no regular pattern of cranial vault deformities, and disorders in the calvaria and orbits represent compensatory alterations secondary to the increased intracranial pressure [44]. For further information about Crouzon syndrome, please refer to Chapter 6.

Apert Syndrome (Acrocephalosyndactyly)

This syndrome is characterized by craniosynostosis, hypoplasia of the midface, symmetric syndactyly of the hands and feet and other axial skeletal deformities, with autosomal dominant inheritance. In association with maxillary hypoplasia, there may be high-arched palate, cleft palate, tooth crowding and anterior open bite, besides choanal atresia [44].

Hypoplasia of the facial skeletal architecture in the three dimensions, especially hypoplasia of the midface, is the craniofacial alteration common to affected individuals [45].

Involvement of the midface is characterized by nasomaxillary and zygomatic hypoplasia, retrusion of the maxillary dental arch and anterior crossbite, often associated with exorbitism [46, 47].

Obstruction of the upper airway is another frequent finding in these individuals, with predisposition to complications as respiratory infections and sleep apnea [48].

Anatomical and functional factors predispose to obstructive sleep apnea syndrome (OSAS) in individuals with syndromic craniosynostosis. The approximate prevalence of 60% in these individuals confirms the increased risk to OSAS in this population compared to individuals without syndromes in the same age range [49].

In addition to these functional aspects, the psychosocial effects caused by the deformities are important factors determining the indication for surgical treatment [50].

For further information about Apert syndrome, please refer to Chapter 6.

Treatment Objectives

Thus, the goal of surgical treatment of facial alterations in individuals with syndromic craniosynostosis is to achieve an outcome that meets correction of skeletal deformities from the functional standpoint, with achievement of facial aspect to allow full social integration of the individual [51].

However, conventional surgical procedures are not indicated in most cases, because even though the characteristic skeletal deficiency in these conditions is three-dimensional, the greater expression occurs in anteroposterior direction and great bone advancements, especially in horizontal direction, are necessary to correct these deformities [50].

Orthognathic Surgery X Surgery for Advancement of the Midface

Conventional orthognathic surgery is best indicated after advancement of the midface when the goal is to accurately correct the occlusion, since in most cases advancements with Le Fort III osteotomy or mono-bloc frontofacial advancement do not allow adequate correction of malocclusion [52].

Similarly, conventional facial advancement surgeries without association of distraction osteogenesis provide only spatial rearrangement of bone segments, without new bone formation and consequent remodeling of the three-dimensional skeletal structure [53]. Thus, facial advancements by Le Fort III osteotomy and mono-bloc frontofacial advancement, associated with distraction osteogenesis, are the procedures of choice for advancement of the midface in individuals with syndromic craniosynostosis [46].

Le Fort III Osteotomy

This comprises advancement of the midface with mobilization including the inferior 3/4 of the orbits, nose, zygomatic bones and maxilla, and is indicated for individuals presenting maxillary hypoplasia with type III facial pattern and Angle Class III malocclusion. Advancement of the midface provided by Le Fort III osteotomy aims at increasing the anteroposterior dimension of the nasopharyngeal airway and reestablishing adequate dental occlusion, besides enhancing the craniofacial esthetic aspect (Figs. **9.9-9.11**) [44].

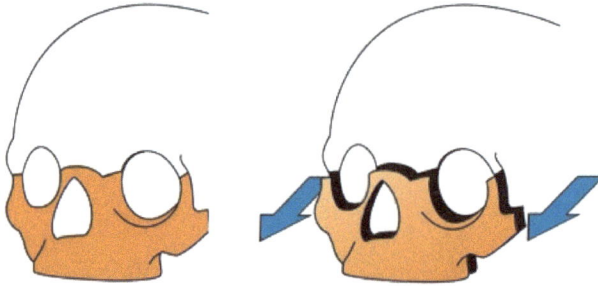

Fig. (9.9). Line of Le Fort III osteotomy used for the treatment of individuals with severe hypoplasia of the midface.

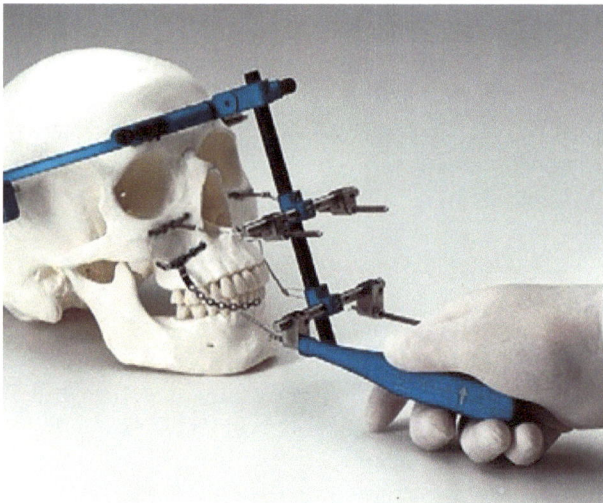

Fig. (9.10). Rigid External Device (RED) employed for distraction of the midface in individuals submitted to Le Fort III osteotomy. Source: KLS Martin, Germany.

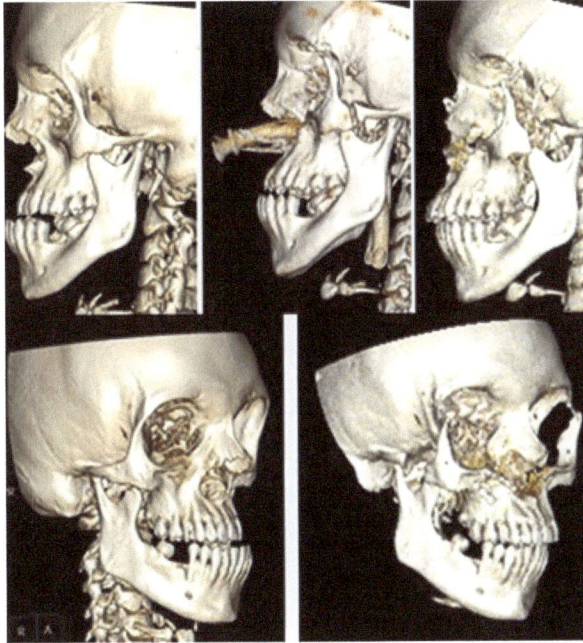

Fig. (9.11). Individual with Crouzon syndrome submitted to Le Fort III osteotomy and distraction osteogenesis of the midface with utilization of RED. Notice the progressive correction of occlusion on the three-dimensional reconstructions of serial computed tomograms of the face during facial advancement.

Mono-bloc Frontofacial Advancement

The mono-bloc advancement comprises simultaneous advancement of the forehead, orbits and midface, being indicated for children with retrusion of the midface, respiratory disorders, exorbitism and corneal exposure. Similar to Le Fort III osteotomy, the mono-bloc advancement aims at reestablishing the craniofacial esthetics, besides increasing the anteroposterior dimension of the nasopharynx. Also, it promotes correction of exorbitism, consequently protecting the cornea (Figs. **9.12** and **9.13**) [44].

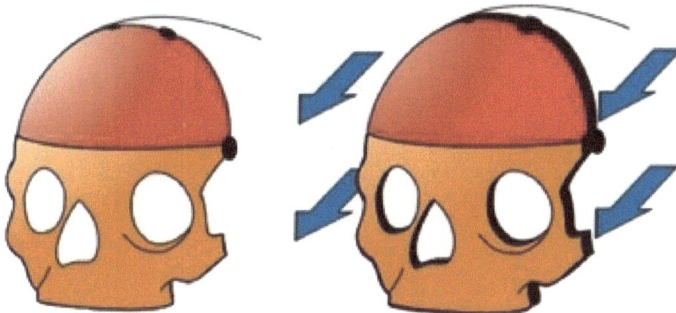

Fig. (9.12). Osteotomy lines of mono-bloc frontofacial advancement.

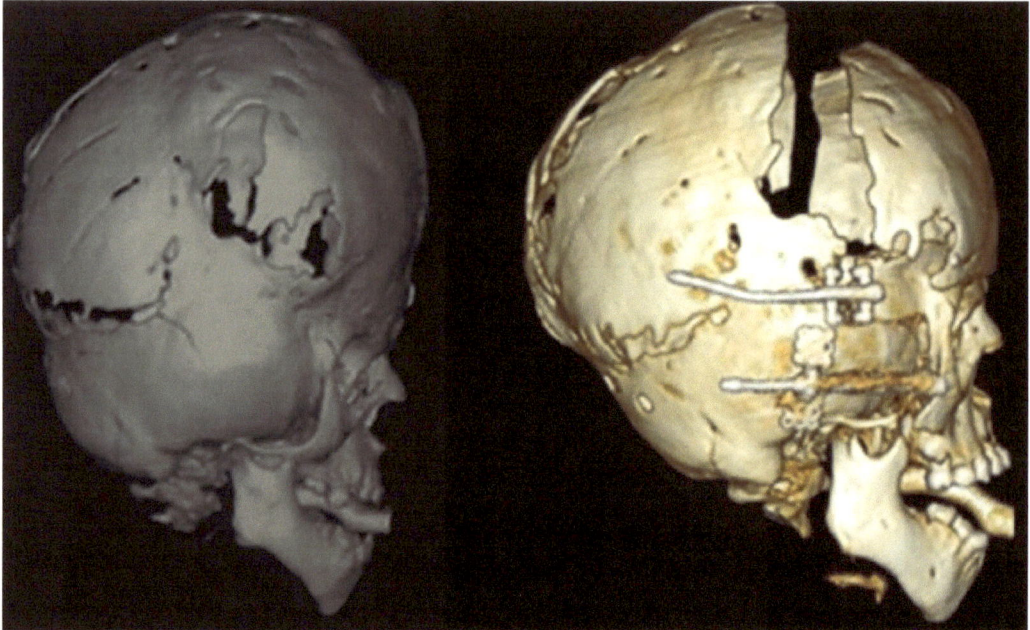

Fig. (9.13). Three-dimensional reconstructions in individual with Apert syndrome, submitted to mono-bloc frontofacial advancement, in this case with utilization of internal distractors.

CONCLUSION

In the presence of large hypoplasias of the facial segments, especially mandibular hypoplasias and hypoplasias of the midface, the traditional treatment methods (*e.g.* Le Fort I osteotomy) are unable to provide satisfactory esthetic and functional outcomes. Distraction osteogenesis is the procedure of choice, minimizing or correcting great hypoplastic deformities, yet without achievement of an accurate occlusion, in which several cases require orthognathic surgery in the future to achieve satisfactory relationship between the bone bases (maxilla and mandible).

CONFLICT OF INTEREST

The author (editor) declares no conflict of interest, financial or otherwise.

ACKNOWLEDGEMENTS

Declared none.

REFERENCES

[1]   Aronson J. Experimental and clinical experience with distraction osteogenesis. Cleft Palate Craniofac J 1994; 31(6): 473-81.
[http://dx.doi.org/10.1597/1545-1569(1994)031<0473:EACEWD>2.3.CO;2] [PMID: 7833340]

[2]   Ilizarov GA. The tension-stress effect on the genesis and growth of tissues: Part II. The influence of the rate and frequency of distraction. Clin Orthop Relat Res 1989; (239): 263-85.
[PMID: 2912628]

[3]   Ilizarov GA. The tension-stress effect on the genesis and growth of tissues. Part I. The influence of stability of fixation and soft-tissue preservation. Clin Orthop Relat Res 1989; (238): 249-81.
[PMID: 2910611]

[4]   Polley JW, Figueroa AA, Kidd M. Principles of distraction osteogenesis in craniofacial surgery. In: Lin KY, Ogle RC, Jane JA, Eds. Craniofacial Surgery: science and surgical technique. Philadelphia: W. B. Saunders Company 2002; pp. 163-71.

[5]   McCarthy JG, Schreiber J, Karp N, Thorne CH, Grayson BH. Lengthening the human mandible by gradual distraction. Plast Reconstr Surg 1992; 89(1): 1-8.
[http://dx.doi.org/10.1097/00006534-199289010-00001] [PMID: 1727238]

[6]   Cohen SR, Rutrick RE, Burstein FD. Distraction osteogenesis of the human craniofacial skeleton: initial experience with new distraction system. J Craniofac Surg 1995; 6(5): 368-74.
[http://dx.doi.org/10.1097/00001665-199509000-00007] [PMID: 9020716]

[7]   McCarthy JG, Stelnicki EJ, Mehrara BJ, Longaker MT. Distraction osteogenesis of the craniofacial skeleton. Plast Reconstr Surg 2001; 107(7): 1812-27.
[http://dx.doi.org/10.1097/00006534-200106000-00029] [PMID: 11391207]

[8]   Mulliken JB, Kaban LB. Analysis and treatment of hemifacial microsomia in childhood. Clin Plast Surg 1987; 14(1): 91-100.
[PMID: 3816041]

[9]   Robin P. Glossoptosis due to atresia and hypotrophy of the Mandible. Am J Dis Child 1934; 48(3): 541-7.

[10]   Robin P. La chute de la base de la langue considerér comme une nouvelle cause de gene dans la respiration naso-pharyngienne. Bull Acad Natl Med 1923; 89: 37-41.

[11]   Sher AE, Shprintzen RJ, Thorpy MJ. Endoscopic observations of obstructive sleep apnea in children with anomalous upper airways: predictive and therapeutic value. Int J Pediatr Otorhinolaryngol 1986; 11(2): 135-46.
[http://dx.doi.org/10.1016/S0165-5876(86)80008-8] [PMID: 3744695]

[12]   de Sousa TV, Marques IL, Carneiro AF, Bettiol H, Freitas JA. Nasopharyngoscopy in Robin sequence: clinical and predictive value. Cleft Palate Craniofac J 2003; 40(6): 618-23.
[http://dx.doi.org/10.1597/02-044] [PMID: 14577814]

[13]   Grabb WC. The first and second branchial arch syndrome. Plast Reconstr Surg 1965; 36(5): 485-508.
[http://dx.doi.org/10.1097/00006534-196511000-00001] [PMID: 5320180]

[14]   Poswillo D. The pathogenesis of the first and second branchial arch syndrome. Oral Surg Oral Med Oral Pathol 1973; 35(3): 302-28.
[http://dx.doi.org/10.1016/0030-4220(73)90070-4] [PMID: 4631568]

[15]   Ohtani J, Hoffman WY, Vargervik K, Oberoi S. Team management and treatment outcomes for patients with hemifacial microsomia. Am J Orthod Dentofacial Orthop 2012; 141(4) (Suppl.): S74-81.
[http://dx.doi.org/10.1016/j.ajodo.2011.12.015] [PMID: 22449602]

[16]   Werler MM, Starr JR, Cloonan YK, Speltz ML. Hemifacial microsomia: from gestation to childhood. J Craniofac Surg 2009; 20 (Suppl. 1): 664-9.
[http://dx.doi.org/10.1097/SCS.0b013e318193d5d5] [PMID: 19218862]

[17]   Passos-Bueno MR, Ornelas CC, Fanganiello RD. Syndromes of the first and second pharyngeal arches: A review. Am J Med Genet A 2009; 149A(8): 1853-9.
[http://dx.doi.org/10.1002/ajmg.a.32950] [PMID: 19610085]

[18]   Cohen MM Jr, Rollnick BR, Kaye CI. Oculoauriculovertebral spectrum: an updated critique. Cleft

Palate J 1989; 26(4): 276-86.
[PMID: 2680167]

[19]   Heike CL, Hing AV. Craniofacial Microsomia Overview. Available at: http://www.ncbi.nlm.nih.
       gov/pubmed/20301754

[20]   Rollnick BR, Kaye CI, Nagatoshi K, Hauck W, Martin AO. Oculoauriculovertebral dysplasia and
       variants: phenotypic characteristics of 294 patients. Am J Med Genet 1987; 26(2): 361-75.
       [http://dx.doi.org/10.1002/ajmg.1320260215] [PMID: 3812588]

[21]   Gorlin RJ, Cohen MM Jr, Hennekam R. Branchial Arch and Oral Acral Disorders. In: Gorlin RJ,
       Cohen MM, Hennekam RC, Eds. Syndromes of the Head and Neck New York. Oxford 2001; pp. 790-
       8.

[22]   Tuna EB, Orino D, Ogawa K, *et al.* Craniofacial and dental characteristics of Goldenhar syndrome: a
       report of two cases. J Oral Sci 2011; 53(1): 121-4.
       [http://dx.doi.org/10.2334/josnusd.53.121] [PMID: 21467824]

[23]   Posnick JC, Ruiz RL. Treacher Collins syndrome: current evaluation, treatment, and future directions.
       Cleft Palate Craniofac J 2000; 37(5): 434.
       [http://dx.doi.org/10.1597/1545-1569(2000)037<0434:TCSCET>2.0.CO;2] [PMID: 11034023]

[24]   Posnick JC, Tiwana PS, Costello BJ. Treacher Collins syndrome: comprehensive evaluation and
       treatment. Oral Maxillofac Surg Clin North Am 2004; 16(4): 503-23.
       [http://dx.doi.org/10.1016/j.coms.2004.08.002] [PMID: 18088751]

[25]   Perkins JA, Sie KC, Milczuk H, Richardson MA. Airway management in children with craniofacial
       anomalies. Cleft Palate Craniofac J 1997; 34(2): 135-40.
       [http://dx.doi.org/10.1597/1545-1569(1997)034<0135:AMICWC>2.3.CO;2] [PMID: 9138508]

[26]   Steinbacher DM, Bartlett SP. Relation of the mandibular body and ramus in Treacher Collins
       syndrome. J Craniofac Surg 2011; 22(1): 302-5.
       [http://dx.doi.org/10.1097/SCS.0b013e3181f7df87] [PMID: 21239924]

[27]   Moore MH, Guzman-Stein G, Proudman TW, Abbott AH, Netherway DJ, David DJ. Mandibular
       lengthening by distraction for airway obstruction in Treacher-Collins syndrome. J Craniofac Surg
       1994; 5(1): 22-5.
       [http://dx.doi.org/10.1097/00001665-199402000-00006] [PMID: 8031974]

[28]   Chong DK, Murray DJ, Britto JA, Tompson B, Forrest CR, Phillips JH. A cephalometric analysis of
       maxillary and mandibular parameters in Treacher Collins syndrome. Plast Reconstr Surg 2008; 121(3):
       77e-84e.
       [http://dx.doi.org/10.1097/01.prs.0000299379.64906.2e] [PMID: 18317089]

[29]   Posnick JC, al-Qattan MM, Moffat SM, Armstrong D. Cranio-orbito-zygomatic measurements from
       standard CT scans in unoperated Treacher Collins syndrome patients: comparison with normal
       controls. Cleft Palate Craniofac J 1995; 32(1): 20-4.
       [http://dx.doi.org/10.1597/1545-1569(1995)032<0020:CMFSCS>2.3.CO;2] [PMID: 7727483]

[30]   Waitzman AA, Posnick JC, Armstrong DC, Pron GE. Craniofacial skeletal measurements based on
       computed tomography: Part II. Normal values and growth trends. Cleft Palate Craniofac J 1992; 29(2):
       118-28.
       [http://dx.doi.org/10.1597/1545-1569(1992)029<0118:CSMBOC>2.3.CO;2] [PMID: 1571345]

[31]   Farkas LG, Posnick JC. Detailed morphometry of the nose in patients with Treacher Collins syndrome.
       Ann Plast Surg 1989; 22(3): 211-9.
       [http://dx.doi.org/10.1097/00000637-198903000-00008] [PMID: 2735721]

[32]   Senggen E, Laswed T, Meuwly JY, *et al.* First and second branchial arch syndromes: multimodality
       approach. Pediatr Radiol 2011; 41(5): 549-61.
       [http://dx.doi.org/10.1007/s00247-010-1831-3] [PMID: 20924574]

[33]   Molina F. Mandibular distraction osteogenesis: a clinical experience of the last 17 years. J Craniofac

Surg 2009; 20 (Suppl. 2): 1794-800.
[http://dx.doi.org/10.1097/SCS.0b013e3181b5d4de] [PMID: 19816352]

[34] Molina F. Mandibular distraction: surgical refinements and long-term results. Clin Plast Surg 2004; 31(3): 443-462, vi-vii. [vi-vii.].
[http://dx.doi.org/10.1016/j.cps.2004.03.008] [PMID: 15219751]

[35] Dec W, Peltomaki T, Warren SM, Garfinkle JS, Grayson BH, McCarthy JG. The importance of vector selection in preoperative planning of unilateral mandibular distraction. Plast Reconstr Surg 2008; 121(6): 2084-92.
[http://dx.doi.org/10.1097/PRS.0b013e31817081b6] [PMID: 18520899]

[36] Vendittelli BL, Dec W, Warren SM, Garfinkle JS, Grayson BH, McCarthy JG. The importance of vector selection in preoperative planning of bilateral mandibular distraction. Plast Reconstr Surg 2008; 122(4): 1144-53.
[http://dx.doi.org/10.1097/PRS.0b013e318185d596] [PMID: 18827649]

[37] Shetye PR, Warren SM, Brown D, Garfinkle JS, Grayson BH, McCarthy JG. Documentation of the incidents associated with mandibular distraction: introduction of a new stratification system. Plast Reconstr Surg 2009; 123(2): 627-34.
[http://dx.doi.org/10.1097/PRS.0b013e3181956664] [PMID: 19182623]

[38] Wilkie AO, Morriss-Kay GM. Genetics of craniofacial development and malformation. Nat Rev Genet 2001; 2(6): 458-68.
[http://dx.doi.org/10.1038/35076601] [PMID: 11389462]

[39] Cohen MM Jr. FGFs / FGFRs and Associated Disorders. In: Epstein CJ, Ericson RP, Wynshaw BA, Eds. Inborn Errors of Development: The Molecular Basis of Clinical Disorders of Morphogenesis New York. Oxford 2004; pp. 380-97.

[40] Fragale A, Tartaglia M, Bernardini S, *et al.* Decreased proliferation and altered differentiation in osteoblasts from genetically and clinically distinct craniosynostotic disorders. Am J Pathol 1999; 154(5): 1465-77.
[http://dx.doi.org/10.1016/S0002-9440(10)65401-6] [PMID: 10329600]

[41] Warren SM, Brunet LJ, Harland RM, Economides AN, Longaker MT. The BMP antagonist noggin regulates cranial suture fusion. Nature 2003; 422(6932): 625-9.
[http://dx.doi.org/10.1038/nature01545] [PMID: 12687003]

[42] Di Rocco F, Arnaud E, Renier D. Evolution in the frequency of nonsyndromic craniosynostosis. J Neurosurg Pediatr 2009; 4(1): 21-5.
[http://dx.doi.org/10.3171/2009.3.PEDS08355] [PMID: 19569905]

[43] Warren SM, Longaker MT. The pathogenesis of craniosynostosis in the fetus. Yonsei Med J 2001; 42(6): 646-59.
[http://dx.doi.org/10.3349/ymj.2001.42.6.646] [PMID: 11754148]

[44] Pinheiro Neto CD, Yoshida M, Alonso N. Síndromes com Deformidades Craniofaciais. 2011.

[45] Alonso N, Goldenberg DC, Lima DS, Camara PR, Matushita H, Ferreira MC. Distraction osteogenesis of the midface with rigid external distractors: preliminary experience in two cases. Braz J Craniomaxillofac Surg 2003; 6: 7-12.

[46] Iannetti G, Ramieri V, Pagnoni M, Fadda MT, Cascone P. Le Fort III external midface distraction: surgical outcomes and skeletal stability. J Craniofac Surg 2012; 23(3): 896-900.
[http://dx.doi.org/10.1097/SCS.0b013e31824e2549] [PMID: 22565921]

[47] Shetye PR, Boutros S, Grayson BH, McCarthy JG. Midterm follow-up of midface distraction for syndromic craniosynostosis: a clinical and cephalometric study. Plast Reconstr Surg 2007; 120(6): 1621-32.
[http://dx.doi.org/10.1097/01.prs.0000267422.37907.6f] [PMID: 18040197]

[48] Meling TR, Tveten S, Due-Tonnessen BJ, Skjelbred P, Helseth E. Monobloc and midface distraction

osteogenesis in pediatric patients with severe syndromal craniosynostosis. Pediatr Neurosurg 2000; 33(2): 89-94.
[http://dx.doi.org/10.1159/000028982] [PMID: 11070435]

[49]   Alonso N, Carpes AF, Hallinan MP. Achados Polissonográficos em pacientes com síndromes de Apert e Crouzon. Rev Bras Cir Craniomaxilof 2009; 12: 98-104.

[50]   Lima DS, Alonso N, Camara PR, Goldenberg DC. Avaliação de pontos cefalométricos no alongamento ósseo do terço médio da face em portadores de craniossinostose sindrômica com a utilização de dispositivo externo rígido. Rev Bras Otorrinolaringol (Engl Ed) 2009; 75: 395-406.

[51]   Passos-Bueno MR, Wilcox WR, Jabs EW, Sertié AL, Alonso LG, Kitoh H. Clinical spectrum of fibroblast growth factor receptor mutations. Hum Mutat 1999; 14(2): 115-25.
[http://dx.doi.org/10.1002/(SICI)1098-1004(1999)14:2<115::AID-HUMU3>3.0.CO;2-2]   [PMID: 10425034]

[52]   Ahn JG, Figueroa AA, Braun S, Polley JW. Biomechanical considerations in distraction of the osteotomized dentomaxillary complex. Am J Orthod Dentofacial Orthop 1999; 116(3): 264-70.
[http://dx.doi.org/10.1016/S0889-5406(99)70236-2] [PMID: 10474097]

[53]   Cope JB, Samchukov ML, Cherkashin AM. Mandibular distraction osteogenesis: a historic perspective and future directions. Am J Orthod Dentofacial Orthop 1999; 115(4): 448-60.
[http://dx.doi.org/10.1016/S0889-5406(99)70266-0] [PMID: 10194291]

SUBJECT INDEX

www.ingramcontent.com/pod-product-compliance
Lightning Source LLC
Chambersburg PA
CBHW041728210326
41598CB00008B/813